Care Ethics and Social Structures in Medicine

This book examines the central structures in medicine—medical knowledge, economics, technological innovation, and medical authority—from the perspective of an ethics of care. The author analyzes each of these structures in detail before considering the challenges they present to end of life care. The perspective of an ethics of care allows for a careful focus on how these structures affect the capacity of the health care system to provide the care patients need, on the impact they have on the relationships between patients and caregivers, and on how they affect the caregivers in terms of their own sense of identity and capacity for care. This book offers one of the first focused discussions of an ethics of care across a wide range of social issues and structures in contemporary medicine. It will be of keen interest to advanced students and scholars in bioethics and health care ethics who are interested in these important issues.

Ruth E. Groenhout is the Distinguished Professor of Health care Ethics at the University of North Carolina at Charlotte, USA. She is the author of *Connected Lives: Human Nature and an Ethics of Care* (2004) and co-editor of *Philosophy, Feminism, and Faith* (2003).

Routledge Annals of Bioethics

Series Editors:
Mark J. Cherry
St. Edward's University, USA
Ana Smith Iltis
Saint Louis University. USA

For a full list of titles in this series, please visit www.routledge.com

Care Ethics and Social Structures in Medicine

Ruth E. Groenhout

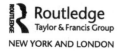

Routledge
Taylor & Francis Group

NEW YORK AND LONDON

First published 2019
by Routledge
52 Vanderbilt Avenue, New York, NY 10017

and by Routledge
2 Park Square, Milton Park, Abingdon, Oxon OX14 4RN

Routledge is an imprint of the Taylor & Francis Group, an informa business

First issued in paperback 2021

© 2019 Taylor & Francis

Library of Congress Cataloging-in-Publication Data
A catalog record for this book has been requested

ISBN: 978-0-367-00022-6 (hbk)
ISBN: 978-1-03-209441-0 (pbk)
ISBN: 978-0-429-44493-7 (ebk)

Typeset in Sabon
by Apex CoVantage, LLC

This book is dedicated to my kids—Ben and Kelsey, Tessa and Caleb, Annemaria, and Gordon—with the hope that they will be enmeshed in structures of care that provide for them for their whole lives.

Contents

Acknowledgments

Portions of this book were written during my time at the Centre for Ethics, Philosophy and Public Affairs at the University of St. Andrews, and I am grateful for the support the Center provided, as well as the sabbatical provided by Calvin College that permitted this effort.

Introduction
Care and Social Structures

The central premise of this book is that an ethics of care offers substantive resources for ethical analysis of contemporary medicine. We are told, regularly, that contemporary medicine is in crisis, whether an economic crisis (Blazheski and Karp, 2018), or a crisis of care (Himmelstein et al., 2018), or a crisis of too few caregivers and too many prospective patients (Kirch and Petelle, 2017; Haddad and Toney-Butler, 2018). But while there is widespread agreement that medicine needs to make changes, it is difficult to know where to begin to think through the complex challenges in a productive way. This book proposes to begin thinking about some of the central issues in medicine by offering a consideration of how a framework developed from within an ethics of care might offer helpful considerations in this process. We do need to think about what the criteria are that we use to evaluate what expenses are too high, or what sorts of care ought to be provided to citizens (or residents of a country, citizens or not), and so on. A basic ethical framework cannot resolve every problem in health care, but it can provide a set of criteria for debating specific issues, as well as a general framework for making decisions about what policies are within a generally acceptable range.

An ethics of care is a theory that makes care central to any consideration of ethical matters, and it seems particularly apt for providing a framework for thinking about contemporary health care practice. This book does not try to provide a complete overview of all the various ethical viewpoints one might consider for such a task, but instead offers an analysis that develops the resources of an ethics of care and considers the potential it offers for thinking about the many challenges we face. And it focuses this analysis on a specific set of issues, namely, the large-scale social structures that structure the delivery of care in medicine today. An ethics of care is a theoretical approach particularly suited to the health care context. It focuses on the relationships that shape our lives and on the social structures that support (or fail to support) those relationships, and it works within a framework that recognizes the fact, so obvious in the context of health care, that people are not equal in power, knowledge, or authority. Physicians and nurses stand in positions of differential authority and power, patients usually don't stand at all, but sit or lie down (visually mapping their situation vis-à-vis those who do stand), and so on. The primary purpose of medicine is care, making an ethics of care particularly apropos for this context. Further, so many good theorists are currently working in an ethics of care framework that the resources it offers in terms of approaching issues from a variety of perspectives is tremendous. Working within an ethics of care framework, then, promises to be a worthwhile method of approaching issues in health care. But much of contemporary medical ethics focuses on individual cases and decision-making by particular individuals. Individual decisions are important, to be sure, but ethical issues in the health care context go far beyond the choices of particular patients or medical professionals.

Because an ethics of care makes caring practice itself central to any ethical evaluation, this provides the over-arching consideration for this evaluation. But just noting that providing care is a good thing doesn't get us very far. This book offers a brief history of an ethics of care, and the methods of evaluation and moral analysis that care ethicists have developed. In the course of that explanation, I will argue that an ethics of care provides resources for evaluating social structures in terms of the following four sets of considerations:

First, how does the structure under analysis provide care, and what sort of care does it provide? In the case of health care, the aim, clearly, is to provide for the restoration of health when possible, to alleviate pain and restore function, to cure illnesses, and so on. But for different types of health care practices, the specifics that define good care will differ. More than this, for the particular structure at issue, the measure of good care will depend on what that structure ought to provide. So, in the case of economic structures, for example, one main consideration, from that perspective of care as well as many other theories will be the question of access—do the economic structures of health care generate an adequate level of access for the population as a whole?

Second, how do these structures fit into the rest of the social systems within which they are contextualized? Economic issues intersect with the development of new technologies, for example, complicating the provision of care and the very notion of adequate access. Likewise, caregivers' authority rests, in part, on their role as gatekeepers for access to health care, and this depends, in turn, on the economic structures.

Third, how do the structures themselves function in terms of providing, facilitating, or obstructing the care that they are designed to offer? This is a central concern for care theory, since relationships of care are, as noted earlier, central to any care analysis. Here the criteria for evaluating better and worse care need to go beyond health outcomes (though clearly these matter) to include the experiences of patients and caregivers alike. Structures that give rise to deep frustrations on the part of caregivers, for example, contribute to burnout and failures of care, and need to be addressed. Structures that make it harder to maintain interpersonal relationships, such as the over-technologization of end of life care, likewise deserve critique.

Fourth, how do the structures affect the capacity of those working within them to actually care for others, and how do they shape the characters of agents in terms of supporting (or destroying, or facilitating, or otherwise affecting) the development of the character traits essential to acting as a caring person? As discussed earlier, the structures within which professionals function shape them in deep and profound ways. The power and authority which accrue to the role of caregiver, for example, are both crucial to the caregiver's job and represent challenges for providing care in situations where patients refuse to accept the caregiver's recommendations.

In Chapter 1 the basic features of an ethics of care that provide the context for this analysis are explained and detailed. The account focuses on the resources of an ethics of care for understanding large-scale structural issues.

The social structures that form the focus of this book are ones that have direct bearing on the provision of care. In Chapter 2, I start with the issue of knowledge and the way different conceptions of knowledge structure the provision of health care. Medical knowledge makes for a particularly interesting case for ethical analysis because the very concept of knowledge has recently undergone a substantial revision, moving from a primarily clinical judgment model to one that bases knowledge claims on evidence-based practice. The shift from clinical judgment to evidence-based practice changes both who is considered an expert and how knowledge is constructed. These changes, in turn, have changed the way that care is given, the standards for what counts as good care, and the self-understanding of caregivers.

Knowledge is not the only structure in medicine that determines the way care is given. In Chapter 3, economic forces and their impact on the provision of care and the character of caregivers are analyzed. In the current politicized climate surrounding economic structures and health care, it is easy to get carried away by rhetoric, proclaiming one's own preferred economic structure to be a moral requirement, one's opponent's to be deeply wrong, evil, and muddle-headed. But my sense is that any economic structure in medicine will have both positives and negatives: some keep costs down more than others, but perhaps at the cost of certain kinds of care. Others may provide a greater range of services, but fail at providing the most basic kinds of care to the most vulnerable, and so on.

Both medical knowledge and medical economics are driven by technological factors. The increasingly sophisticated technology that health care currently offers has changed the delivery of care and the ways that caregivers function. Chapter 4 focuses on the increasingly technological structure of contemporary medical care and the way that technology functions in positive and negative ways in the provision of care.

Knowledge, economic factors, and technology all represent forms of power in medicine. Social structures track this power, for the most part, making those who have the most knowledge, those who control the economics, and those who provide and control access to the technology the ultimate authorities in the medical field. But power and authority are never absolute, and the complexities of modern life are such that knowledge and economic control, or technological control, do not always coincide. So medical practice involves with competing structures of power, and Chapter 5 turns to the complexity of power and authority in the medical context, looking at how it supports (or sometimes frustrates) caregivers.

Finally, Chapter 6 turns to some of the deepest questions in medicine—namely, questions about what the ultimate aims of medicine really are. If we are to care well in the medical context, we need to have some shared sense of what we are trying to achieve when patients come seeking care. But contemporary medicine has some deep conflicts in its understanding of what good care consists in. One place where these conflicts are particularly apparent is in the realm of end of life care, where conflicts between those who argue for fighting against death as long and as hard as possible and those who argue for a good (i.e., painless) death have become quite strident in recent years. These issues get to the heart of what medicine is and ought to be, and of what it means to provide the sort of care that we should ensure for all members of our communities.

An ethics of care is a good fit for thinking about the ethics of health care precisely because of the overlap between many of the central concerns of medicine and the resources offered by an ethics of care. First, care is central to medicine. A famous debate of a number of years ago focused on whether medicine should focus on care or on cure—that is, whether the primary ends of medicine should be assumed to be the correction of conditions identified as diseased, abnormal, or dysfunctional (that is, primarily cure), or whether medicine, while including a concern for curing illness, needed to have a broader focus on care for the whole patient, care that encompassed both cures for illness and care for conditions that either need not be cured (pregnancy and childbirth) or cannot be cured, amelioration of suffering, preventive care, and health promotion. The general consensus today is that medicine encompasses far more than just cures, and it is common to find discussions that advocate for both cure and care (see, for example, De Valk et al., 2001; Glouberman and Mintzberg, 2001), or identifies both as central values in medicine (Giordano, 2018). Medical practice as a whole encompasses more than simply cure, and a single-minded focus on cure can increase patient suffering (Cassell, 1998). Care, then, is the over-arching goal of medicine.

More than this, because patients enter the world of medicine when they are vulnerable, sick, and sometimes dying, what they look for from their caregivers is more than simply diagnosis and prescription of treatment. There is an existential aspect to the medical encounter because patients so often are facing conditions that could either change their lives drastically or signal the end of their life altogether. Caregivers find themselves asked to respond to needs that go far beyond merely the need for treatment of physical conditions; they are asked to provide emotional and psychological support for individuals facing death, or watching a family member die.

While emotional support is possible in these cases, caregivers often cannot fully respond to the deepest existential questions patients pose. These are existential questions, after all, precisely because each of us must face our own death, and that is a burden no one can take from us. While an ethics of care cannot resolve these questions, it provides space for addressing them and recognizing their importance in a medical context.

An ethics of care offers an ethics focused on practices of care, so it is not surprising to find that many care ethics discussions emphasize medical practice as either one central component of care (Engster and Hamington, 2015; Sevenhuisjen, 2004; Tronto, 1994) or as a central focus of their analysis as a whole (Petersen, 2008). Because medicine is a set of practices that provide physical care aimed at protecting health, providing alleviation of suffering, and supporting people's abilities to live well, it is a central part of the care that allows us to live and flourish in the contemporary world. Its central role makes it a natural focus for an ethics of care. Care ethics also has much to offer medicine. It is a theory designed to examine complex relationships of care, one that recognizes the vital importance of the work that goes on in medical facilities, and a theory that emphasizes the centrality of embodiment and the physical world, as well. This book, then, is an exploration of the intersection between these two.

1 Care Ethics and the Practice of Medicine

The problems facing health care in the contemporary world are massive. The costs of health care continue to rise at astonishing rates, technological advances contribute to those spiraling rates, and caregivers find themselves increasingly working in a setting where patient care is compromised, burnout is rampant, and bureaucratic oversight creates serious inefficiencies. But addressing any of these problems on its own seems almost impossible because of the interwoven factors that structure health care in the modern world. Between the complex interactions between insurers, caregivers, patients, and politicians, and the added complexities of clinical research, hospital bureaucracies, alternative medicine, and legal oversight, there are no simple answers to the question of how health care could be reformed.

Nor can this book offer any easy solutions, but it can bring some clarity to the various issues that contribute to the complexity of contemporary health care. If we begin with a focus on the specific issue of care—the care that is provided by doctors, nurses, and other professionals, and supported by a wide range of institutional structures, from insurance companies to hospital administrators, from researchers to lawyers to politicians—and if we keep our focus on what does and does not support the provision of care itself, we will find that the lack of easy answers does not rule out the possibility of thinking in new ways about the provision of health care. So this book examines the big, over-arching structures of health care: knowledge, economics, authority, and technology, and examines them using the perspective of an ethics of care to think through how some of the problematic aspects of those structures might be addressed.

This book brings the resources of an ethics of care to an analysis of central structures in medicine: structures of knowledge, economics, authority, and technology, examining the realm of contemporary medicine through the lens of a care ethics account of relationships and how they function.

This first chapter begins with a brief account of care ethics, its history, and current development. After this very rough sketch, I offer a more specific development of the particular features of an ethics of care relevant to my analysis in this book, identifying the specific aspects of an ethics of care I will rely on in my analysis. The chapter then turns to the question of what I am calling 'social structures in medicine.' The structures I want to identify by this phrase are structures that aren't determined (solely) by intentional policy decisions or identified in consent forms. Instead, what I am interested in are the background structures that function in contemporary medicine—structures that shape the practice of medicine profoundly, but which are not best addressed in terms of individual choice. Some of these practices have changed rather radically in recent decades (the shift from a clinical judgment model to an evidence-based model of medicine, for example). Others change only incrementally (the authority structures in medicine remain largely unchanged, in spite of numerous attempts to move to medical team models and shared decision-making). In the last section of this chapter, I discuss what I am calling social structures in a bit more detail, as well as explain why I have chosen to examine precisely these ones, and some general notes about what an ethics of care perspective brings to an analysis of such structures.

Care Ethics: A Brief Introduction

The ethics of care has its earliest beginnings in the writing of various feminist theorists starting in the 1980s. The term 'ethics of care' itself was coined by Carol Gilligan in her book *In a Different Voice*, a book in which she argued that men and women frequently spoke in 'different voices' in ethics, men tending to use a voice of justice, while women used a voice of care (Gilligan, 1982). By these two terms, Gilligan separated out concerns about rights, principles, boundaries, and protection of autonomy (masculine ethics, using the language of justice) from concerns about relationships, care, emotional bonds, and protection of connections (feminine ethics, using the language of care).

Women's Voices and Practices of Care

Gilligan's book touched off a wide-ranging discussion of ethics, gender, social policy and research methodology that went on for a good two decades. Many theorists found her research problematic (Brabeck, 1993), others rejected the dichotomy between care and justice (Friedman, 1993), and there was intense criticism of her linkage between a particular ethical voice and women (Card, 1995). But she did provide a term for something that clearly resonated with many feminist thinkers. Nel Noddings, in particular, wrote *Caring: A Feminine Approach to Ethics and Moral Education*, in which she argued that traditional ethical theory has consistently excluded women's voices and concerns, and that this exclusion has resulted in a lack of attention to aspects of ethics that are particularly important in many women's lives, namely: emotional connections, relationships, and the provision of care to the vulnerable and needy (Noddings, 1984).

Like Gilligan's work, Noddings' work proved controversial, with critics charging her with naiveté (Koehn, 1998) and with producing an ethics that entrenched patterns of exploitation of women (MacKinnon, 1987). Regardless of the controversy, however, Noddings' work was important for its willingness to speak from a perspective that took the sorts of jobs many women have performed throughout time and across many regions, and examined the way that doing this work might shape one's understanding of ethics.

As care ethics developed, this focus on how practices shape both an individual's capacity to care and their capacity for moral reasoning became a central part of care theory. Sara Ruddick, for example, examined the way that practices of mothering develop epistemic virtues that are crucial for human life. (Mothering, on Ruddick's account, is a practice that both men and women could engage in, but it has historically been a set of tasks relegated to women.) Among these epistemic virtues are attentiveness, knowledge of basic features of human flourishing, and (more controversially) pacifism (Ruddick, 1989). The analysis of practices and their relevance to care ethics has been central for many subsequent thinkers (Myers, 2013; Tronto, 2012; Kittay, 1999) and provides the focus on the sorts of knowledge and emotional habituation that develop with the performance of particular sorts of practices and social roles that I will rely on in this book. Just as mothering can develop skills, habits, and epistemic virtues, medical practices can develop ethical skills and habits, as well as epistemic virtues, that are crucial to the provision of care. But improperly structured practices can do the opposite, and can force practitioners to cease caring and to become emotionally distant and prone to ignore ethically relevant aspects of a situation.

The combination of Gilligan's language of a feminine voice, Noddings' focus on women's experience, and Ruddick's emphasis on mothering meant that early discussions of an ethics of care took place largely under the rubric of feminist ethics and women's issues. While not all theorists who work with an ethics of care are women (this acknowledgment will come as a relief to Lawrence Blum, Michael Slote, and Maurice Hamington, I imagine), all take women's experiences seriously because of the centrality of what is often called care work to both women's experiences and the development of care ethics. Michael Slote goes so far as to consider the possibility that women are naturally more ethically gifted than men (Slote, 2007, p. 71). The more common position in care ethics has been that the social roles women tend to play generate the sort of caring concern and attentiveness that ground ethical responsiveness more generally (Noddings, 1984, 1989; Held, 1993, 2006; Hamington, 2004). Because particular social roles and types of work provide training in care work, then, and care work provides the context for an analysis of care more generally, care work and related practices have been a central focus of care ethics.

Care work, loosely defined, is the work done to provide care for others, particularly the care that is needed to take care of bodily needs, but also the work needed to develop and sustain basic capabilities in the other (Tronto, 1994; Engster, 2007). It includes such practices as mothering (or parenting—there is some debate over what the better term is), elder care, daily activities such as housekeeping, cleaning, and cooking, and a wide range of other activities. All of these provide for central needs in human life, all require repetition and continuous re-doing of the work, and all tend to receive very low payment, if those performing them are paid at all. The specific sort of care this book focuses on is health care: the care work that attends to health needs of individuals and populations, provided by professionals (for the most part) in systems organized socially to provide medical care and health support services to a population. This socially structured provision of care is a central concept in nursing theory (Watson, 2012; Boykin and Schoenhofer, 1993; Bishop and Scudder, 1991). It has been less prominent as a theoretical component of medical ethics, though it is a vital part of medical practice, as indicated by the way that medical practice is regularly referred to as medical care, and those who provide it as caregivers.

Care work requires a set of habits and practices that are central, care theorists have argued, for the ethical life. Attentiveness (for example, the capacity to see that a toddler is uncomfortable because he needs to go to the bathroom), the willingness to notice that a sticky counter needs to be wiped off, or the recognition that an elderly client is suffering from an unusual level of dementia, straddles the boundaries of epistemology and ethics because it is both a matter of knowledge and a matter of will. One has to care about another to be fully attentive, but one also has to process the information that comes from caring. In addition to attentiveness and understanding, care work also requires imaginative development, as noted by Maurice Hamington and Rita Manning (Hamington, 2004; Manning, 1992). The development of an embodied imaginative awareness of another's situation, in particular, is a crucial part of care in general, and a vital part of the caring work that goes on in the medical field (Vosman, 2017; Halpern, 2001). These epistemological capacities and skills cannot be developed simply by reflection. They are, as Hamington emphasizes, embodied skills, developed through engagement in specific practices of care. The capacity to engage in them is damaged when the social structures one inhabits trains one to ignore or become insensitive to another's needs or suffering, and can be virtually destroyed when one engages regularly in practices that inflict damage or harm on others. Practices of care generate skills that one needs time to acquire, and performing caring work well requires practice and imaginative engagement.

Because of the ways that caring practices shape a person's character and generate epistemological capacities for recognizing what care requires, engaging in care practices shapes one's character and perspective on issues in important ways. Among them, as Sarah Ruddick and Eva Feder Kittay have noted, is the capacity to see connections among people—Ruddick argues that mothering can be the basis for a politics of peace, while Kittay argues that seeing all people as 'some mother's child' fundamentally changes one's attitude toward strangers and others (Ruddick, 1989; Kittay, 1999).

In both cases, the connections are not deterministic (mothers can support war efforts, and mothers can also be pretty brutal toward other people's children), but connections nonetheless exist. One might note in this context the extent to which women have been portrayed as insufficiently 'principled' to be truly ethical precisely because they do tend to care about the lives and suffering of other people's children. As Kant puts it: "I hardly believe that the fair sex is capable of principles. . . . But in place of it Providence has put in their breast kind and benevolent sensations" (quoted in Mahowald, 1994, p. 105). Far nobler the masculine willingness to kill than the feminine proclivity to pardon, in his view.

Rejecting the simplistic gender essentialism that prompts the Kantian claim, we can still note that there are clear correlations between providing care and being capable of seeing and responding to the specific needs of who and what are cared for. Caregivers tend to have a fairly realistic sense of the nature of those cared for, what they need to flourish, and what nuances of behavior indicate problems. Whether we are considering plants, dogs, patients with Alzheimer's, or second graders, those who work with them day in and day out are most likely to have practical wisdom about the best way to meet their needs and help them flourish; they are also more likely to pursue other policies that protect the standing of those they care for. Elementary teachers vote for the political party they think will preserve money for education, gardeners tend to support land preservation policies, and so on. There is, of course, an element of circularity in this account—providing care for the vulnerable makes one particularly capable of seeing the need for care, and of seeing what care requires—but the circularity is not vicious, but rather akin to Aristotle's notion that the person who becomes virtuous knows more about what virtue requires than others. The development of practical wisdom requires practice.

Health care work, however, generally requires more than just practice in caregiving. Health care is a specialized field of knowledge, one that requires extensive education, whether one is a physician, a nurse, or a technician of one type or another. The practical wisdom developed by good caregivers is more than just wisdom developed by experience. It is grounded in highly technical understanding of human physiology and the various methods of responding to health and illness. Because of this, caring in the health care context depends crucially on the social structures that make that knowledge possible, and on the systems of health care provision developed to make the provision of care possible and effective. These social structures and systems themselves, then, are essential parts of the provision of care, and deserve careful analysis in terms of their capacity to provide the care they are intended for.

Providing care is an essential part of human life, particularly the child care without which the species would cease to exist. One would expect that the sort of work I have been describing as care work, both private and professional, might get more respect than it does precisely because of its centrality to human existence (Held, 1993). It hasn't, however, and the lack of attention to care work in philosophy seems to be over-determined by a large number of factors. Philosophy has historically been considered the province of men. Though women have obviously contributed, their voices are relatively few and far between, and frequently erased from the subsequent history (McAlister, 1996; Lerner, 1993). But it is not just women's presence that is erased from Western philosophy. Entire areas of life that are relegated to spheres associated with women (whether the 'private' or the 'domestic' or issues involving children or the education of the young) are either treated as not philosophically interesting, or simply ignored as being outside the realm of important parts of human life (Okin, 1979; Elshtain, 1981; Nye, 1988). Philosophers in the past who have focused on issues of the education of young children, such as Plato and Rousseau, generally advocate protecting them from the pernicious effects of their female caregivers so that the more rational males can educate them properly (Green, 1995).

So, women's voices are marginalized and erased, and the areas associated with them are ignored or criticized, rarely treated as areas where expertise relevant to philosophical thought might be found. The modern legacy of this traditional blindness is a general tendency for philosophers to simply fail to see that an account of human nature that ignores care work is lacking an important component, or to assume without reflection that matters pertaining to children or the elderly are simply irrelevant for general ethical theorizing. As Virginia Held notes, discussing the practices of child care:

> That this whole vast region of human experience can have been dismissed as 'natural' and thus as irrelevant to morality is extraordinary. It may be outside moralities built entirely on abstract rationality, modeled as these are on an abstraction of the supposed 'public' realm. But that only shows how deficient these moralities are for the full range of human experience.
>
> (1993, p. 36)

The development of an ethics of care, then, is in part a very deliberate attempt to develop an ethical theory that attends to the full range of human lives, from birth to death, as it is experienced by both caregivers and care receivers, and as it is experienced by actual embodied humans rather than disembodied rational egos or abstract calculating machines.

A word is probably in order here about the notion of essentialism. So far, I have spoken of women's voices, of the social practices that are largely relegated to women, and the like. I am speaking in generalities here—obviously, some men have engaged in practices of care, and the voices of the women that entered philosophical conversations in earlier generations were almost exclusively women of the upper class with extraordinary privilege and few caregiving responsibilities. Critics of an ethics of care have frequently pointed to such issues in charging care ethics with an incipient essentialism. According to such critics, care ethics mistakenly attributes certain types of characteristics to women on the basis of their sex, and assumes that it is somehow a part of women's nature to act and feel in certain ways, and so on.[1]

But as has been pointed out numerous times, the recognition that certain tasks are socially allocated to women (or to men) hardly requires an essentialist position. Further, recognizing that the social position (whether privileged or not) that a woman (or a man) occupies is likely to have an effect on her perspective is also not essentialist (Hartsock, 1999). One might also point out that paying attention to the way that social groups are positioned with respect to socially powerful roles is a central part of feminist theory, as the large number of anti-essentialists who have resorted to 'strategic essentialism' in order to continue to advocate for women's rights suggests (Stone, 2004). In any case, since the question of essentialism is not central to the focus of this book, and since a care ethics analysis does not need to take a stand one way or another on the issue, for my purposes here I will assume that the capacity to care is an essential human attribute, but not necessarily a gendered one, and that one's capacity to care is developed by engaging in practices of care on a regular basis. Women's caring activities, thus, are relevant to, but not definitive of, caring practices. Any account that ignores them, however, is an incomplete moral theory. This also indicates another reason why care ethics is particularly important for thinking about health care. Many discussions of medical ethics assume that ethical matters in medicine involve physicians (a stereotypically masculine role) and patients. The central role of nurses in the practice of medicine is strangely absent from many analyses. An ethics of care offers a perspective from which to rectify this omission.

Care and Empathy

Because an ethics of care focuses on the character traits, epistemological skills, and capacities such as attentiveness developed by practices of care, an ethics of care will have more in common with virtue accounts of ethics than with either a rationalist/deontological or a universalist consequentialist conception of ethics. While rational deliberation is an important component of ethical practice, from an ethics of care standpoint, the use of rationality will not require the squelching or erasure of emotional responses. On the contrary, an ethics of care has clear connections to the many historical figures (Hume, Aristotle, Augustine) who emphasize the centrality of emotions to the moral life, and a number of feminist theorists have noted these connections (Baier, 1994; Nussbaum, 2001; Groenhout, 2004; Slote, 2007). The particular emotions connected with practices of care, such as empathy, love, and the concern evoked by observing vulnerability in another, are clearly central to an ethics of care: Nel Noddings considers these the natural basis upon which an ethics can be built (Noddings, 1984). Other theorists such as Michael Slote consider empathic caring to be the central feature that makes a response truly moral (Slote, 2007). Nursing theory has also noted the importance of both intellectual and affective components of good care (Bishop and Scudder, 1991) and some theorists in medicine have likewise noted the necessity of empathetic responses for good care (Halpern, 2001) and the ways that the structures of medicine can make caring difficult (Brody, 1992).

Empathy is the capacity to feel with another, to recognize and resonate with another's emotions. It is clearly a necessary condition for the sort of moral response care ethics makes central to ethics, since anyone incapable of recognizing another's emotional state will also be incapable of caring about what the other is feeling and responding appropriately. As mentioned, Slote considers empathetic caring to define moral obligation. "[A]ctions are morally wrong and contrary to moral obligation," he writes, "if, and only if, they reflect or exhibit or express an absence (or lack) of fully developed empathic concern for (or caring about) others on the part of the agent" (Slote, 2007, p. 31). On his account, it is the intentional state and its emotional basis that generates moral rightness or wrongness.

Other theorists, among whom I would classify myself, adopt an account of caring that acknowledges the central role empathy plays in ethical motivation without making it the determining feature of an ethics of care. In part, this debate reflects differences in the focus of analysis. When analyzing actions, an idealized empathic care offers a reasonable standard for evaluating the nature of the action. But in evaluating social structures, empathy is less useful for several reasons. One is that social structures are not generated or sustained purely by individual decisions, but are instead created and maintained in part by inattention and habit. They pre-exist the individual and take on a sort of life of their own that is sometimes immune to what individuals would choose if they could. The question of whether they are conducive to providing good care cannot be resolved by asking if those working within them exhibit empathic care, but must be investigated in terms of the actual effects of the structures for the provision of adequate care for health-related concerns.

Another reason why empathy is less useful for evaluating social structures is that the shape of the social structures themselves sometimes determines what counts as an empathetic response. In a society that provides little in the way of elder care, for example, caring children, acting out of empathy, would presumably do their best to care for their aging parents. But in a society with broad social support networks, the same actions might be evidence of an attempt to control one's elderly relatives, and might not be a properly empathetic response at all. But if what can count as an ideally empathetic response is dependent on the social structures, it becomes difficult to use the test of idealized empathy as the measure of ethical acceptability.[2]

Empathic caring, then, is of interest insofar as it is supported or impeded by the social structures under analysis, but it is not, in and of itself, the central focus of the analysis. Because I am looking at broad-scale social factors, the focus in this book will be on the ways that social structures affect the capacity of practitioners to offer empathetic care, on the ways that the systems function smoothly (or badly) when providing health care, and the like. Analysis of these systems requires attention to the shape and nature of the practices that make up the health care system.

Caring Practice

Practices can be roughly defined as ongoing participation in socially constituted and socially coordinated activities. Caregiving and the development of the capacity to care both occur in the context of practices—most usually, though not always, practices of care. Such practices can be as mundane as walking the dog or as sophisticated and complex as the care provided in a contemporary intensive care unit (ICU), but they are properly considered practices of care if their primary focus is that of caring for the basic needs of others. Practices of care operate within social contexts that constitute the criteria for acceptable and unacceptable care, they require shared social meanings about the nature of human life, and they are often the location where a culture instills its basic worldview and unspoken assumptions (Bishop and Scudder, 1991).

Caregivers and care receivers, then, are defined (and often define themselves) largely in terms of the social meanings and values of the cultural context within which they take place. Because of this direct connection to the social settings within which they acquire meaning, caregivers and care receivers are best thought of as porous selves, as human beings whose sense of self and identity are profoundly relational and dependent on others. Rather than framing this as an automatic negative, care theorists consider it a basic aspect of human identity, one that needs to be recognized in theories of autonomy (Mackenzie and Stoljar, 2000) for example, or of rationality (Code, 1991). After all, if human selves are porous, the fiction of an isolated ego capable of some form of pure rationality untouched by social context cannot offer an adequate account of the nature of human thinking, and certainly will be inadequate when it comes to an account of moral reasoning.

Because a focus on caring practices draws attention to the social contexts within which care is given and human lives experienced, social structures are an essential part of the moral terrain that care theorists are concerned with. Specific social structures analyzed have ranged from elder care (Tronto, 1994) to care for people with severe mental disabilities (Kittay, 1999) to the care work that makes the development of healthy children and healthy citizen relationships possible (Held, 1993; Ruddick, 1989). In focusing on the structures that function in the provision of care, these theorists reject the standard boundaries between ethical theory and social/political theory, since the provision of care in society involves both individual actions (and intentions) and broader social structures. Consider, for example, Held's discussion of raising children.

Caring for children, Held notes, requires a complex set of individual intentions, emotions, and choices. Parents know that taking care of children, both when they are small and as they grow, is a complex and difficult task, one that requires both intellectual abilities and emotional attachments. It also requires a depth of practical wisdom about the structures of social life—without this one cannot parent well since part of parenting is preparing a child to survive and (ideally) flourish in the social context they will inhabit. But the individual parent doesn't function in a vacuum. She or he engages in the care work of parenting in the context of social structures that profoundly influence the nature of the care itself. She may be raising a daughter in a rigidly patriarchal society; he may be raising daughter in a country that is structured so that women are presumed to be the primary caregivers. She may be raising an intersexed child in a culture that requires her to check one of two boxes for 'gender' on every doctor's chart and school form; he may be raising three kids with inadequate funds while trying to hold down two minimum wage jobs. Given the social nature of care, one cannot analyze practices of care without paying attention to the many ways that social structures set the context within which care is given, and in some cases even define what care can be.

Care theory, then, begins with the recognition that humans are irretrievably social beings, that our existence, our identity, and, a fortiori, our ethics, needs to be analyzed within a social framework. Further, that social framework is dependent on the provision of care for its very existence. Humans need care at most points in their lives, but they cannot survive without care at a number of significant junctures. Infancy and childhood are obvious cases, as are the many times when we face serious illness, disabling conditions, or other types of vulnerability. At each of those points in our lives, we depend on others to care for us, often in a way that precludes absolute reciprocity, while depending on a general willingness to participate in general structures of care. By absolute reciprocity I mean the ability to repay care received with care given to the specific agent who provided care in the first place. Generally, this is not how care works; those who receive from one person often give back to others and some who receive care never provide care in return, some because they are incapable, others because they are freeloaders, others because the mobility of the modern world takes them far away from their initial caregivers, and so on.

So, human life involves a circulating system of care provided and received by a wide variety of agents, sometimes provided informally (as when friends help each other out), or formally but without economic arrangements (as when parents care for their children), or as a matter of paid employment (as when an in-home aide cares for an elderly individual, providing meals, cleaning services, and personal assistance). The recognition that this is the basic structure of human life also tells us something about human nature—that humans are beings who care, and that care is fundamental to their lives as humans.

Further, care theory has identified a number of features of healthy caring relationships that are important for understanding the dynamics of social structures in health care delivery. One follows directly from what I have just referred to as the circulating system of care. Caring relationships are characterized by reciprocity, by a mutuality of care given and received by both parties to the relationship. But the reciprocity is what Selma Sevenhuisjen, following Iris Marion Young, terms an asymmetrical reciprocity (Sevenhuisjen, 2003). Rather than a contractual sense of reciprocity in caring relationships whereby the care one receives is returned either in kind or in comparable value, the care given and received can be quite disparate. Caregivers in a health care setting provide extensive services for patients, and there is no expectation that the patients return that care directly to them, even if that were possible. But patients and their families do respond to care, both by accepting the care as directed toward their good, and by responding with gratitude for good care. One of the reasons noncompliant patients are difficult to deal with is that they respond to treatment that is meant for their good as if it were either unimportant or actively malevolent, and that response makes the relationship one that is hard to sustain.

It is not the case, however, that all the responsibility for proper responsiveness to care falls on the patient (or the patient's family). As Noddings noted in her initial articulation of care, the one who receives the care completes the act of caregiving, in a way, by giving evidence that the care is recognized as good (Noddings, 1984). But in some cases, what the caregiver offers as care is not experienced as good or as caring. In such cases, it can be appropriate for the one receiving care to point out that what is being offered is not meeting his or her needs. We will see the social structure version of this dialogue later in this book in discussing the development of hospice in response to patients who rejected the overly technological, overly interventionist treatments that had become standard treatment for end of life cases.

In recognition of the centrality of both affective responses and practice in caregiving, care ethics is closely related to a virtue ethics—requiring agents to act in ways that develop the capacity to care, that develop the skills needed for competent caring, and that develop feedback loops to ensure that what one intends is what the other receives (since one person's attempts at care can be experienced by another as unbearable interference, and the like). Care ethics provides us with a set of habits, skills, and epistemological requirements that we need to develop if we are to be truly caring people. This is among the reasons why care theorists reject a simplistic dichotomy between reason and emotions—good caring requires rational reflection, and reason cannot function properly without the development of certain emotional capacities, as well as certain value judgments.

Becoming a caring person does not happen in a vacuum, however. Which individuals need or can be provided care, the shape of that care, and appropriate venues for engaging in care are all socially contextualized. Joan Tronto, Nel Noddings, and Virginia Held have all argued that an ethics of care requires that we pay attention to the social conditions under which care is offered (Tronto, 1994; Noddings, 2002; Held, 2006). I have argued for this same point, and consider it a central aspect of an ethics of care (Groenhout, 2004). There are several reasons why an exclusive focus on just the individual's character fails to provide an adequate moral analysis.

The first reason comes from the complicated interactions between individual character and social context. It is a good thing to work to become a caring moral agent, but if that work goes on in the midst of deeply unjust social structures, and one is not engaged in combatting that injustice, the care one provides may support the injustice rather than challenge it. Diemut Bubeck makes this point in a critique of Noddings' early work (Bubeck, 1995), noting the role that care can play in maintaining (or combatting) systems of injustice. As an example, consider recent shifts in the diagnosis and treatment of depression. While in the past it was frequently assumed that women are just naturally prone to depression and should be medicated when presenting with symptoms, contemporary treatment of depression has become far more aware of the role that social conditions, particularly physical and emotional abuse, can play in triggering depression. Caring psychiatric responses require more than just providing medication that enables an intolerable situation to be tolerated.

A second reason why care needs to be situated within a broader social analysis is that what counts as caring behavior will vary from one context to the next. The debates over end of life care indicate this context dependency. For ordinary medical treatment, offering a range of treatments and exploring options with a patient represents a standard level of good care. In the context of end of life care, however, where the burdens of heroic treatment may outweigh any minimal extension of life, and where many normal patients' response of denial makes evaluating treatments difficult, discussing treatment options needs to be handled with a far greater level of sensitivity and care in explanation. The context changes the way treatment options should be explored.

A third reason why care needs to incorporate a social structure analysis is that any adequate ethical theory needs to do more than address personal motives and character. As humans, we are capable of thinking outside the circle of our own family interests, and responsible moral agency requires that we do so. Reflection about the structure of society, about the way we organize our lives together, is an essential part of a fully human life. In the context of care, then, caring as a full human being requires that I examine the ways that care provision fits into social systems that are themselves either supportive of (or destructive of, or neutral toward) providing care. The employer-provided private insurance model of providing health care for many people in the US, for example, is a system that makes the provision of care enormously complicated in any number of ways. The system was not set up to get in the way of care; private insurance was devised in order to facilitate care. But the combination of a complex health system, third-party payers making coverage decisions, and employer-provided coverage supplemented with an array of government programs for the provision of care has resulted in a bewildering bureaucratic mess.

Care analyses often focus on the difficulties faced by individual agents, whether family members, professionals, or patients trying to negotiate this system, but in this book, I am more interested in what an ethics of care can provide in terms of analyzing the system itself. This is a project that has been addressed by theorists such as Daniel Engster and Joan Tronto at the level of government policies (Engster, 2007; Tronto, 2013), and their analyses will be important for much of what I have to say. But the focus in this book is not on government policies, for the most part, so much as it is on how specific social structures in the health care context function to support or impede the provision of care.

Obviously, policies set at a national level are relevant to many of the social structures of contemporary health care, and this will be addressed at various points. But the focus of this analysis is on how the structures that exist affect the capacity to provide care in concrete ways. For example, American health care is largely provided through a system of private insurance, creating the need for care providers to negotiate with specific corporations when trying to gain access to care for patients. Faced with an insurance company unwilling to cover needed treatment, individual caregivers are often forced to choose between shading the truth (aka, lying) or failing to provide adequate medical treatment, an obvious moral dilemma. It is important to think about how caregivers can deal with such issues; but it is perhaps more important to spend time reflecting on how we might avoid such dilemmas going forward by changing the system that generates the problem. Joan Tronto's analysis of the way that elder care is provided, and the ways that women's unpaid care labor has contributed to a system that lacks a universal system of elder care (Tronto, 1994), is one exemplar of this type of analysis. The point of such an analysis is not to somehow accuse those doing the hard work of caring for the elderly of doing something wrong; it is rather to recognize that the whole of a particular system may produce something quite opposed to the intentions of individual participants.

Specific Features of Care Ethics Relevant to Analysis of Social Structures

Several features of a care ethics analysis that are clearly relevant to any analysis of social structures have already been mentioned and, in some cases, discussed at some length in this chapter. First, the centrality of care as an emotional response is clearly relevant in a number of different ways. Although I will not assume that empathetic care determines the moral valence of what is analyzed, it is certainly relevant to any analysis.

Actions, decisions, and policies that are generated from motives that are contrary to or in opposition to care and empathy are problematic on any account of care ethics. In what follows I will assume that decisions that (for example) take a terrible toll on the physical and psychological health of patients for the sake of relatively minor financial benefits for a health care institution are clearly worthy of criticism. Caring professionals do not trade off patient welfare for minor financial gain.

A second way that empathetic care will structure this analysis is via a concern about the effects of particular practices in terms of the sorts of people the practice produces. Theorists such as Alastair MacIntyre have noted that practices necessarily shape character (MacIntyre, 1984), and from a care perspective, this shaping represents an issue worth paying attention to. Once a professional is inculcated into a practice, the daily activities and structure of the profession itself can turn the professional into a person she or he does not really want to be, a person who cannot easily provide the sort of care she or he ought. The challenge for our moral development is more frequently that of thinking about how structures that are not designed for systematic dehumanization, but instead designed to provide care, might still produce extremely problematic changes in people's character because of structural features that aim at generally good goals.

An example helps to show how this can happen. Nursing is an occupation that places care at the very heart of its identity. Acute care nurses work in a setting that is designed to provide care to some of the most vulnerable and needy members of our society. One would expect that acute care nursing, then, would be a social structure that shapes practitioners into the sorts of people with the characteristics that most enable their particular area of caring practice.

However, the contemporary health care scene is characterized by extreme concerns for efficiency. In nursing, the result has been that the patient population in the acute care setting is, overall, sicker and more acute than would have been the case 30 years ago (as is a result of increasing use of outpatient surgery, etc.). At the same time that patients need more care, staffing numbers have been cut, exacerbating the demands on the nurse's time. While good nursing programs still promote holistic health care and teach nursing students to care about the full range of patient concerns (emotional, spiritual, social and physical), in practice, many nurses find that they barely have time to give adequate physical care to patients (Poncet et al., 2007; Aiken et al., 2002). Spending time talking about the patient's emotional response to the news that they have pancreatic cancer and that it is inoperable is extremely difficult, sometimes impossible.

Worse, when nurses find themselves heavily over-scheduled, patients who do need extra care, whether because they are difficult for emotional reasons, or simply not responding well to a particular treatment protocol, can generate resentment and frustration on the part of their caregivers. Facing too many, too-sick patients, a nurse is likely to respond to demanding patients with anger rather than support, though good nurses recognize this temptation and work hard to defuse it. It is, however, a natural outcome of being over-scheduled and knowing that all of one's patients face serious health issues; extra time given to one patient comes out of the care given to others, and that means the demanding patient is taking time away from others who are as or more needy.

This is an unhealthy dynamic. (Do I really need to say this?) Nurses are the sorts of people who want to care, so when they have to work in a situation where they are forced to give sub-par care, they face a difficult conflict between their own sense of identity and their actions on a daily basis. They deal with this in a variety of ways. Some nurses simply give up and become relatively uncaring functionaries (to their patient's detriment), though my sense is that these are relatively infrequent cases and often miserably unhappy people. Other nurses struggle to maintain their basic identity under conditions that make it very difficult for them. Many simply give up—high rates of burnout in the nursing profession have been linked, in part, to the increasingly efficient and mechanical structuring of nursing practice itself (Abellanoza et al., 2018; Munnangi et al., 2018).

This is a case where a legitimate aim in health care (efficiency) is implemented in such a way that it does serious harm to the sense of self of a group of practitioners who are absolutely vital to the over-arching goal of medicine. Efficiency is not evil in and of itself, and it is a crucial component of any sustainable health care system. But calculations of efficiency are usually conducted in terms of hours worked, procedures performed, and medicines distributed—it is almost unheard of for them to include time spent actually talking to patients about what they are frightened of, or how well they understand what their diagnosis is, or simply how they are doing. These latter conversations tend to be seen as inefficient uses of time, in spite of the fact that they are a central component of nursing care. So long as this conflict remains, and so long as efficiency is used as the sole measure of proper functioning in a hospital setting, nurses will continue to experience a serious conflict between their identities and the way they have to work.

When efficiency becomes the standard by which nurses are evaluated, the structure of health care delivery can undermine the character that health care workers should have. If nurses remain in their jobs, they are almost forced to become people who don't care, who perform their tasks efficiently but with no room for occasional extras of time and attention (Monsalve-Reyes et al., 2018). The structure of acute care nursing, in this respect, undercuts—and sometimes destroys—the very characteristics nurses need to be able to really care for their patients.

As I hope is clear from this example, social structures that are problematic from a perspective of care need not be designed to undercut care; in many cases, they are designed to support or provide care. Efficiency, after all, is an important part of any sustainable health care system. Nor need they result from bad motivations or evil intentions. But the structures themselves create patterns of behavior that are not what they should be and that not only make it hard for nurses to act in caring ways; they make it hard for nurses to be caring people.

The character traits I am particularly interested in here cover a range of attributes. Good care requires some obvious characteristics: attentiveness, responsiveness, and good judgment are all obvious (and widely discussed in the literature). Patience, gentleness, and honesty all play a role, too. When social structures are well ordered, these characteristics are supported or encouraged by the context within which people conduct their care work; when social structures are badly ordered, the opposite occurs. In many cases, the structures may be relatively neutral with respect to the virtues carers develop. While not optimal, this is also not necessarily bad and may not be worth changing, given the potential costs—foreseen and unforeseen—of large-scale social change.

One of the central principles that informs this analysis, then, is that social structures ought to facilitate both the provision of good care and the development and sustaining of caregivers' capacity to provide care. In the context of health care, the measurement of good care is context dependent, since the type of care being offered (palliative care, psychiatric care, primary care) determines in large part what constitutes good care. I will be assuming, for the most part, that the actual measurement of what constitutes good care can be evaluated by assessing such features as health outcomes, patient satisfaction, and the other sorts of outcomes that are central to the sort of health care being offered.

Caring outcomes themselves, and the effects of social structures on the capacity to care, will be two of the central lenses through which social structures will be analyzed. Two other features of care ethics will also be relevant to this analysis. The first is access to care, and the second is the issue of relationships of care. In speaking of access to care, I move from one meaning of care (emotional motivation) to another (meeting someone's basic needs), meanings that frequently blur in the context of discussions about an ethics of care. The blurring occurs for a reason, since the emotional response of care naturally produces the activities that meet another's needs (though not in every case), and the activities themselves are frequently received as expressions of the emotional motivation. Nonetheless, the two do differ, and can be discussed separately (Hamington, 2004).

So, when I speak of access to care in this context, I am speaking of the specific types of medical care that are available in the contemporary world: professional diagnoses, pharmaceuticals, surgical interventions, and skilled nursing care. An ethics of care focuses our attention on the ways that such care is provided, and the various ways that social structures can facilitate or impede access. While emotional caring is one important aspect of an ethics of care, the fulfillment of people's health care needs is also relevant, and separate from the motivations of the caregivers.

Finally, this analysis will focus at points of what I will call relationships of care: the networks of interpersonal connections within which people live and understand their lives. As discussed earlier, people's sense of self and understanding of how they act or are treated are structured by the networks of social meanings within which they exist. These networks of meanings and social understandings, then, are crucial for making sense of a wide range of issues in health care. In order to make sense of structures of authority in medicine, for example, we need to see how self-understandings of physicians depend in crucial ways on the way that patients respond to them (Mohrman, 1995). Part of what makes being a physician a high-status profession in the contemporary world is the gratefulness and respect with which patients respond to doctors. This is appropriate in certain ways, because the care offered by physicians is so important for so many reasons, but it can also generate problems when a physician's sense of self becomes too tied up with a sense of authority so that any challenges or questions are seen as attacks on his or her very sense of self. Without an understanding of how interpersonal relations function, however, thinking through what sorts of authority are appropriate and what sorts are problematic, becomes difficult.

Social Structures and Care

The social structures discussed in this book are of various sorts. In subsequent chapters, I will be discussing the structure of knowledge, economic factors in health care, the nature of authority, and the role that technology plays. All of these interact in complex ways, so the discussion of any one will of necessity connect to discussion of others. One cannot discuss the conceptualization of knowledge in medicine without also considering the relationship between authority and expertise, for example. Likewise, the way that knowledge claims are structured has economic ramifications; decisions about what treatments will be covered in many insurance plans is frequently a matter of whether a particular treatment has been shown to be effective, as determined by particular conceptions of knowledge production. While physician opinions as to effectiveness were considered authoritative in years past, for example, today the preference is for large-scale statistical analyses.

But all of these issues share some common features. First, they are social. All are parts of human communal reality, and exist as parts of practices and actions cooperatively engaged in by large numbers of people over large amounts of time. They are all, then, both entrenched and difficult to change, and, simultaneously, generated by human decisions and actions. Further, as with many social structures, so long as we are enmeshed within them, they tend to seem natural and automatic. It is only when they change, or when we switch vantage points, that we can focus on the social structure itself, rather than simply take it for granted as the necessary background of action.

A second aspect that is worth noting is the way that these various social structures create the context within which many ethical questions and quandaries arise. To take one example, it is because medical treatment is considered a scientific enterprise aimed at staving off death as long as possible that medical technology has become both so efficacious and so expensive. Were we to have the perspective on medicine offered by Socrates in Plato's

Republic, that the best medicine either cures one quickly or lets one die (406e), presumably we would think very differently about the proliferation of technological responses to various medical conditions. We would also, presumably, take a very different approach to questions about how health care systems should function economically, and so on. The importance of these contextual matters, however, is often omitted from medical ethics discussions that focus on individual cases, largely because they fade into the background and are simply assumed rather than examined.

All of the structures that form the focus of this book, however, have become contentious for one reason or another in recent years. The move to implement evidence-based practice has made contentious the question of what counts as knowledge in medicine, while the soaring health care costs facing American citizens have forced our attention to economic structures. Debates about patients' rights, new professional positions such as nurse practitioners and physician's assistants, and an increasing demand for professional recognition on the part of nurses has led to challenges to the structure of medical authority, and so on. And when questions about these sorts of issues are raised, they require a different sort of analysis than many have offered of other issues in medical ethics.

Imagine, for a moment, the case of a single-parent father with young children, holding down two low-paying part-time jobs to keep the family afloat. If one of his children comes down with a serious illness, the social structures within which he lives generate a whole series of difficult ethical questions that seem to have no good answers. As a caring parent, we will assume, he wants to provide good care for his child, but the care he can give is severely compromised by the social situation in which he finds himself.

One of the structures that constrains his condition is economic, obviously. Wages for hourly workers have not kept pace with increases in cost of living for the past 30 years, effectively requiring people to work more hours just to meet minimal needs. While we can debate the pros and cons of government intervention (or lack thereof) into the relationship between employee and employer, there is no denying the fact that the less people are paid per hour, the longer they have to work to make enough to survive, and this has a clear impact on their ability to care for their children. So, our hypothetical father needs to work long hours in order to provide for his children's basic needs, but working long hours will require that he leave a seriously ill child in another's care for lengthy periods of time. Further, caregivers are rarely equipped to care for severely ill children. Our father may not be able to find any caregiver willing to take his child on, and without some form of child care, he cannot maintain his jobs. Working long hours also makes it very difficult to get a child in for treatment in any regular way; clinics are often open only during business hours, and taking time off work may not be possible if he wants to keep his job.

Further, as many health care systems try to move toward a model of health care that treats patients (and families) as those who are primarily responsible for their own health issues, our hypothetical father may find that he is being asked to bear too much responsibility for choices he does not have the expertise to make. While it is, on balance, a good thing to encourage informed and responsible patients, an already overwhelmed parent with too much on his plate may not find this responsibility bearable, and he certainly will find it difficult to do the sort of research that may be necessary to figure out what treatment models may best work for his sick child. Trying to function as a patient advocate for his child, without the time, energy, or resources necessary to play that role adequately, is likely to lead to despair and frustration.

The purpose of medicine is care—for the sick, the vulnerable, those in pain, and the dying. The modern world has an extensive network of systems to provide these types of care, some of which work almost miraculously well, others of which are seriously dysfunctional. Medical ethics textbooks are full of examples of the latter, difficult ethical case studies that prompt students to try to figure out what the correct ethical response is to some heart-wrenching difficulty faced by a patient or a nurse or a physician. But in the case of the father we are considering, it is not so much his individual decisions that need to be examined; it is the context within which care is provided for his sick child.

The social structures of medicine can make the provision of care more difficult, in some cases, or they can support or enhance the provision of care. While one might expect that all of medicine would be structured so as to provide care, the contingencies of a number of factors (the historical structuring of professional relations, interactions with other social structures, sheer bureaucratic inertia) have produced structures that can impede the provision of good care. Further, while care is the central purpose of medicine, there are enough other complicating factors in the contemporary health care context to sometimes make caregivers feel that the last thing they are able to provide is care. My goal, then, is to get a clearer sense of how the various structures in contemporary health care function in terms of making care more or less accessible, in terms of necessary trade-offs between various aspects of care provision, and in terms of how the structures impact the character of the caregivers. And, finally, the analysis will also note that there is often no easy way to restructure problematic aspects of caregiving. Changing structures to address one set of concerns often generates a whole new set of problems that may be as damaging to the provision of care in their own way as the prior problems were in theirs. Care theory emphasizes the particular over the universal in part because it recognizes that many ethical responses need to be local and partial rather than abstract, universal, and overly simplistic.

Notes

1 It is surprisingly hard to find feminist authors who unqualifiedly criticize Noddings as essentialist. The claim that such criticisms are standard occurs widely, so

perhaps it was a very common claim in informal discussions of care ethics, without, being made in print. For an excellent discussion of 'essentialism' in feminist theory more generally, interested readers should turn to Cressida Heyes' 1997 article, "Anti-Essentialism in Practice: Carol Gilligan and Feminist Philosophy" *Hypatia* 12(3): 142–163.

2 This is, obviously, not a complete argument, and I would expect that theorists such as Slote would have responses available to them. These considerations are offered to indicate why a theorist might make something other than empathy central to her analysis.

2 Medical Knowledge
From Clinical Judgment to Evidence-Based Practice

Contemporary health care has awesome resources for responding to health issues. Considering what is known today about, say, the treatment of cancer, compared to what was known just 75 years ago, generates the sense that one is looking at two completely different worlds. Contemporary medicine is a powerful force in the world, in part, because of the amount of knowledge it has generated—about various conditions, about how treatments work, about the best approach to many issues—and it clearly has the potential to continue to provide new insights.

At the same time that the knowledge available in health care has multiplied, the nature of that knowledge and what constitutes it has become more complex. Medicine faces questions about who should be considered an expert, about what constitutes knowledge, and about why some certainties in health care (pregnant women should not drink coffee) remain prevalent in spite of the lack of evidence while others (ulcers are caused entirely by stress) have changed profoundly in response to new evidence. Questions about the nature of knowledge and evidence, while clearly more prevalent in philosophical circles than in medical circles, have become quite important in the contemporary medical context.

The importance of these questions has been driven, in part, by a profound shift in the way that medical knowledge is conceptualized in Western medicine over the past 30 years or so. In the past, medicine was characterized as an art, one that was science-oriented and learned, to be sure, but an art nonetheless. As an art, medical knowledge was understood primarily in terms of clinical judgment, the capacity of the skilled practitioner to identify and treat complex and subtle medical problems. Contemporary medicine, in contrast, aspires to a scientific model of knowledge, and has adopted an account of knowledge based on the paradigm of evidence-based practice (EBP[1]). I am going to draw the distinction between these two models quite sharply at the beginning of this chapter, because in the abstract, the two models offer very different pictures of what counts as knowledge and who can claim the authority of being a knowledgeable practitioner. I'll then complicate the picture slightly, since in practice the distinctions are not as sharp or as clear as purely theoretical considerations might suggest (Parker, 2005; Karthikeyan and Pais, 2009). Setting up these two models will allow us to think about how they function in terms of shaping the practice of health care, however, and will allow for an analysis of both from the perspective of an ethics of care.

Throughout this book, I will be examining alternative models of various aspects of medicine: knowledge in this chapter, economics in the next, technology in the one after that, and so on. In each case, my goal is to avoid a simplistic analysis that holds up one model as the good one (the caring one) while disparaging the other as the bad one (ooh! Uncaring!). My sense is that human life is complicated, as are the demands of care, and one goal in this book is to untangle some of those complications in ways that allow a richer understanding of what is at stake when we change (or choose not to change) the social structures of health care. So, this chapter will not argue that the move to EBP is a mistake, nor will it argue that the clinical judgment model needed to be discarded. Instead, I will argue that both models offer strengths and weaknesses, and that the switch from a clinical judgment model to an evidence-based model has produced both positive and negative results in terms of how care is delivered.

Current debates in health care reflect this complexity. Proponents of clinical judgment argue that EBP can generate 'cookbook' medicine, practitioners trained in following the steps in decision-tree protocols without the trained judgment that the older model required (Groopman, 2007). Defenders of EBP note that it includes clinical judgment as well as patient values in the very definition of evidence that it encompasses, and point to significant improvements in standards of care brought about by the move to EBP (Sackett et al., 2000). Both are correct. There are important strengths of the clinical judgment model that an ethics of care should recognize (its attention to particularity, its recognition of the need for training in practical judgment), while it also carries with it some baggage that is problematic from the perspective of an ethics of care (its hierarchical nature, for example). Likewise, EBP offers important positive characteristics (lessening of hierarchy, accountability, increased accuracy) while also running the risk of creating new problems (blind spots, a tendency to over-privilege pharmaceutical remedies, and some diminishment of clinical judgment skills). Health care knowledge is complex and requires the integration of extensive factual knowledge, psychological insight, and practical wisdom, and any overly simplified account of knowledge will get some of the details wrong.

But while it is vital to recognize that any account of knowledge will need to be nuanced and carefully worked out, it is also important to note that the focus of these different models of knowledge does produce important structural changes in the way health care professionals are trained, in their methods of practice, and in their ability to claim authority. These issues will be the focus of the analysis of this chapter.

Two Paradigms: Clinical Judgment and Evidence-Based Practice

As mentioned earlier, the picture drawn in this section is a bit over-simplified. In actual practice, the lines between a clinical judgment model of medical knowledge and an EPB model are not so clear. But the two models do adopt very different paradigms for the ideal case of knowledge, and it is those divergent paradigms that I focus on here.

Clinical Judgment

On the traditional, clinical judgment account, medicine was thought of as closer to a craft or an art than a science (in the sense of contemporary experimental science). There are a number of reasons for this. One is that physicians care for single patients and make individualized diagnoses, while experimental scientists study whole populations in order to produce statistical generalities. The main goal of a physician is the good of the individual patient, while the goal of an experimental scientist is the generation of knowledge. On this model, the physician uses the results of science to generate a body of knowledge, but the art of medicine requires the application of those general rules to a particular case. This focus on the particular and the unique requires practical wisdom rather than generalized knowledge.[2]

The development of good clinical judgment depends primarily on one particular skill: an experienced practitioner's capacity to see and recognize aspects of a patient's condition that go beyond a mere listing and ranking of symptoms and tests. The notion of judgment (as opposed to calculation) is central to the notion of medicine as an art because it establishes a space for an experienced practitioner to rely on prior experiences, unconscious cues, and expert knowledge in coming to an understanding of what sort of condition the presenting patient has.

Over the course of the development of modern medical education, the clinical judgment model shaped the training physicians received in numerous ways. Many of the components of clinical judgment were codified as part of the development of medicine as a professional practice, as well. Four features of clinical judgment, in particular, deserve our attention:

1. *Training and Experience*: Traditionally, one learned how to be a doctor primarily by working with doctors. Medical education, on the traditional model, was divided into the first few years of classes to provide the background knowledge needed for medicine, after which the students would enter clinical training in a residency program. The residency component of medical education occurs in hospitals or clinics, and provides opportunities for the resident to observe how various techniques are done, and then try to perform them under the supervision of more experienced doctors. Traditional medical education was

thus split between a period of intense theoretical study during which the student accumulated background factual knowledge, and residency whereby practical judgment was developed and trained by a combination of modeling and practice.

The period of residency is a formative time in a physician's career for developing diagnostic skills and learning treatment protocols. While doctors are expected to regularly attend continuing education, these courses need not (and often do not) involve hands-on practice in new techniques. So, one of the results of the way that medical education is structured is that most physicians have learned, and are most comfortable performing, techniques in use in the hospital at which they were residents, at the time when they went through residency. For a number of conditions, however, treatment protocols have changed drastically in (say) the last 20 years, though older doctors often continue using the same techniques they were originally trained in. This results in a certain level of inertia in treatment protocols, since new protocols may be developed, and be shown to be effective, but if they aren't familiar, many doctors won't implement them. And, obviously, this will vary from health care system to health care system, since some are quite proactive about expecting physicians to update their practices, and others not so much.

2. *Diagnostic Judgment*: When medical students are being trained to be doctors, they don't just learn techniques. They also learn how to diagnose what is wrong with someone, a skill that is difficult to learn and requires a fairly lengthy period of training and observation. Many patients come in for treatment with similar sets of complaints—they don't feel well, their lungs are congested, and they have a fever, for example. Sometimes a patient with these symptoms has a cold or the common flu, and other times something much more serious: tuberculosis or pneumonia, for example. Learning the art of diagnosis involves recognizing subtle cues that distinguish these various conditions.

Students, of course, learn the basics of identifying diseases during the years when they are taking course work. But knowing, in theory, what the signs of a particular disease or health condition are is very different from being able to identify that disease or condition when a person has it. The problem is that very few cases of disease look just like the textbooks say they should, or progress just as the textbooks describe. Textbooks describe general rules, while individual cases don't follow the rules, as anyone who has ever tried to find anatomical features in an actual animal or cadaver (as opposed to a textbook or computer diagram) finds out very quickly. The textbook may say that pneumonia characteristically involves a fever. But this patient may not have a fever at all, and may still have pneumonia. A doctor has to learn to recognize patterns of symptoms, minor and not easily characterized differences between conditions, and eventually, to really just see that this is one condition rather than another.

This is one of the keys to good clinical judgment—learning to see patterns in a patient's symptoms, and using those patterns to figure out what the patient does or does not have. Doctors often talk about the gestalt of clinical judgment. What they try to learn to do is to see the whole picture rather than just a list of individual symptoms, and learn a framework of patterns that make sense of the symptoms. An experienced doctor, then, can use clinical judgment to make quick, accurate diagnoses of very vague symptoms—this is one central aspect of good clinical judgment.

3. *Physiological Mechanisms*: In spite of the earlier distinction I made between science and art, medicine does not set itself up as a matter of purely individual intuition in the diagnosis and treatment of various conditions. Instead, it has defined itself since early days as an art informed by science. Stefan Timmermens and Marc Berg argue that one of the hallmarks of clinical judgment is a reliance on pathophysiology. "[D]iagnostic and therapeutic reasoning," they write, "relates symptoms and interventions to the underlying pathophysiological mechanisms that the physician infers to be taking place in the patient's body" (Timmermans and Berg, 2003, p. 88). Research on clinical reasoning bears out the importance of understanding the causal mechanisms, although they also note that this is more pronounced in the case of researchers than practitioners (Patel et al., 1999). This is an important part of the physician's claim to authoritative knowledge. One of the reasons that standards are so high for medical schools, and the curriculum is so rigorous, is the assumption that understanding physiological mechanisms is vital for good clinical judgment.

As I will discuss later, nurses also develop diagnostic skills, and make clinical judgments, but in the early years of modern medicine, their role involved the expectation that they would defer to the judgment of physicians. (This expectation has changed in the contemporary world for a number of reasons, and these changes have complicated the authoritative structures of medicine in ways I will discuss in a later chapter.) The physician's absolute authority in traditional medicine was justified by appeal to the physician's greater degree of understanding of the physiology of the disease and the way that the proposed treatment would interact with the patient's physical condition. And this leads directly to the ways that the clinical judgment model incorporated a very strongly hierarchical model of medical authority in general.

4. *Authority and Hierarchy*: There are very strong hierarchical expectations built into both medical education and the structures of medical decision-making. In traditional programs, residents are expected to

submit to the authority of the attending physicians, and first-year residents are to submit to third-year residents. Further, overt challenges to the authority of anyone further up the food chain are treated as serious disciplinary problems. For the most part, this is a system that works well. Given the huge body of knowledge that physicians need to master during their years of training, and the years of experience of those teaching them, and the constraints of time (particularly in an acute care setting), obedience is generally the most expedient and safest response in any given situation.

At the same time, however, when too rigidly enforced, this strong hierarchical structure can also have problematic effects: elderly physicians can require residents to use outdated treatments, residents required to submit can fail to learn skills of patient advocacy, and patients (who occupy the lowest rung on the hierarchy ladder) can feel alienated and infantilized.

These are the four features, then, that provide us with a somewhat oversimplified picture of medical knowledge as developed in a clinical judgment setting. On this model, medical knowledge claims rested on the twin pillars of practical experience (in both treatment and diagnosis) and physiological knowledge, and were incorporated into a strongly hierarchical system of authority and power. The evidence-based model is designed quite specifically to provide a very different model of both training and practice, coupled with the claim that an alternative model can better reach the central goal of medicine: the well-being of the patient.

Problems with the Clinical Judgment Model

While the clinical judgment model has a number of strengths, it also has some serious weaknesses. The argument for EBP, in fact, specifically identifies several ways that the clinical judgment model fails to protect the best interests of the patient. First, EBP's advocates argue that a shift to an evidence-based system will generate better outcomes for patients because it offers a self-correcting system. According to proponents of EBP, the clinical judgment model virtually ensures that many patients will be treated with out-moded and sometimes detrimental treatment protocols. Further, they argue, the clinical judgment model works well when those at the top of the power hierarchy are truly excellent, but when they are mediocre or (in the worst case) incompetent, the clinical judgment model makes it almost impossible to challenge their decisions. Consider just a few scenarios that are familiar to anyone who spends much time in a health care setting:

Scenario one: a patient presents in a teaching hospital with symptoms that are vague, but consistent with either a serious (but relatively rare) condition or a common and not-terribly-serious condition. The resident, who is unsure of her diagnostic skills, spends considerable time with the patient, going over her case and her test results carefully, and comes to the conclusion that the patient has the serious condition. An overworked and busy attending comes by, briefly eyes the chart, and insists that the patient be treated for the unserious condition. And the resident is too scared to stand up for her original diagnosis because of concerns about challenging authority (remember that hierarchy plays an important role in this model). So, the wrong treatment is given and the patient suffers.

Scenario two: a patient is in the last stages of dying from pancreatic cancer, and her doctor is offering little more than the same pain medications that he has been prescribing for the last 20 years. Even though several new generation pain meds are available, he isn't really familiar with how they work or when they are appropriate, and so chooses to use only what he knows. The nursing staff are horrified at the pain the patient is suffering, but don't feel that they can challenge the authority of the attending, and no other doctor wants to get involved in the case.

Both of these cases are relatively commonplace occurrences, and both represent sub-standard care. And both are direct results of built-in features of the clinical judgment model. Clinicians who have been fortunate enough to practice under truly skilled instructors are likely to have really good diagnostic skills, but those trained under mediocre physicians are unlikely to rise much above their teachers. And, unfortunately, the laws of statistics remind us that at least half of all clinicians will be worse than average when it comes to any set of clinical skills. The clinical judgment model has no built-in way to separate out the good clinicians from the mediocre ones, and its emphasis on seniority and hierarchy make it likely that there will be significant numbers of mediocre practitioners dictating how all those beneath them practice medicine.

Second, because there is no intrinsic mechanism for critical self-examination, the clinical judgment model offers no pressure on clinicians to regularly upgrade or update their knowledge and skills. The weight of tradition, in fact, makes it very difficult to introduce new treatments and change established practices, precisely because the model places so much emphasis on experience rather than alternative sources of knowledge. Further, because the one major source of scientific knowledge in the clinical judgment model is the understanding of physiological processes, physicians will tend to trust treatments that seem to have obvious physiological mechanisms. Traditional treatments generally have been justified, over lengthy periods of time, by reference to some physiological mechanism or another, and while some of these are accurate, others are not. But the mere existence of a mechanism that can be cited is like to make clinicians loathe to try an alternative treatment, particularly one that does not have an obvious physiological justification.

Evidence-Based Practice

What EBP offers is a structural solution to situations such as these, by defining medical practice in terms of "the integration of the best research evidence with clinical expertise and patient values" (Sackett et al., 2000, p. 3). In order to accomplish this, evidence-based practice holds out the following as central components of skilled medical practice.

1. *Research, Literature Searches, Large-Scale Studies*: EBP advises practitioners to base treatment decisions on research. As might be guessed from the name, evidence-based practice defines knowledge in terms of whether or not one's conclusions are based on evidence. If evidence relevant to diagnosis, treatment, or complications is available, then decisions must be based on that evidence in order to count as knowledge. If evidence is not available, then the practitioner needs to recognize that knowledge is lacking. Critics sometimes claim that EBP rejects clinical judgment altogether, but proponents argue that clinical judgment is one source of evidence, a source that should be used in tandem with the best evidence available from clinical studies. Clinical judgment is thus demoted somewhat, since it is no longer the highest standard for knowledge. Along with de-emphasizing practiced judgment, then, EBP emphasizes literature searches and the knowledge generated by clinical research. One standard introduction to EPB, in fact, is titled *How to Read a Paper*, indicating the centrality of literature searches to this model of medical knowledge (Greenhalgh, 2010). In effect, this locates medical authority in the body of research generated by medical studies, rather than in the individual practitioner's diagnostic skill and clinical judgment.

2. *Best Practices*: A second central feature of EBP is an emphasis on learning to analyze statistical data pertinent to treatment decisions, and to base diagnoses and treatments on that statistical data (Howick, 2011). Even when a treatment is one that a doctor has never used, EBP says the doctor should use it if the evidence suggests it has a better outcome than other treatments. This is, again, a significant departure from the clinical judgment model of medicine, in which practitioners generally trust their own experience and observation more than they trust reports of alternative treatments. In effect, an EBP-trained physician is likely to tell a patient, "Well, I haven't used protocol X on this condition, but it has the best outcomes and fewest side effects, so I think we should try it," while the clinical judgment-trained practitioner is more likely to say "Protocol X is being used by many for your condition, but I haven't seen how it works, and I've seen really good results from protocol Y. I'm more comfortable recommending Y because I know how it works."

EBP emphasizes statistical studies that generate data about which treatments produce the best outcomes, overall, and then trusting that data when making treatment decisions. It does not emphasize learning pattern recognition so much as learning to calculate the probability that these symptoms correlate with a particular condition. As new information is added (through lab tests, or through watching the development of the patient's condition), these probabilities will change, but the argument is that doctors are less likely to make mistakes if they rely on hard evidence and probabilities rather than primarily clinical judgment. Further, practitioners are expected to conform to what the data show to be the best practices, rather than making decisions based on their own observations and experience.

Reflecting this approach to medical decision-making, some health care systems have moved to computerized patient charts with standardized questions into which various symptoms or conditions or test results can be entered. Although almost all of these computerized models have the potential for entering data that is outside the parameters, studies have shown that the extra work of 'thinking outside the box(es)' serves as a powerful disincentive; most physicians simply check appropriate boxes and move on. At its worst, this model generates what critics disparagingly call 'cookbook medicine': treating symptoms as little more than boxes in a decision-making tree, and treatment decisions as simply a matter of trying the first protocol on a list of possibilities, then moving to the next in sequence if the first doesn't work out. At its best, EBP ensures that patients get the best treatment for their condition, rather than less-effective treatments that a clinician happens to be familiar with.

3. *Outcomes-Based, Not Explanation-Based*: While medical students are still expected to learn vast reams of physiology and biochemistry, EBP models do not emphasize this aspect of medical knowledge. Instead, EBP emphasizes outcomes, not explanations: what is important, on this model, is whether or not something works. Research need not demonstrate why a treatment works in order to be relevant. Not only does EBP emphasize using treatments that work, whether or not the underlying physiological mechanism is understood, EBP also advocates *not* using treatments if they cannot be shown to work.

It is important not to overstate this difference from the clinical judgment model, of course, since understanding the pathophysiological causal mechanisms of a patient's condition is important for making treatment decisions whether one emphasizes clinical judgment or evidence-based practice, but there is an identifiable difference in emphasis here that can lead to disagreements between practitioners. One area where this disagreement can be seen is in the revision of treatment for peptic ulcers. In the past, it was assumed that excess acid was the cause of peptic ulcers. This seemed to be a clear case where the physiological mechanism causing the ulcer was understood, and the treatment recommendations responded to that understanding. In the mid-1980s, however, Warren and Marshall argued that ulcers were caused by bacilli, and should be treated with antibiotics (Malfertheiner et al., 2009). The results of their proposed protocols were clearly better than the prevailing treatments (and they went on to receive the Nobel Prize for Medicine and

Physiology for their work in 2005). But what was interesting about the episode was the debate in medical circles that occurred immediately after their research appeared. It was not clear when Warren and Marshall's work first appeared *why* a bacterial infection would generate ulcers. The bacteria they had identified (now called *Helicobacter pylori*) are present in many people, yet caused ulcers only in some. And there are ulcers that are not caused by H. pylori (most notably an increasing amount caused by low-dose aspirin regimens and other non-steroidal anti-inflammatory drugs [NSAIDs]). But the treatment Warren and Marshall advocated did get results, even though the exact mechanism of the bacterial cause of the ulcers wasn't known. The shift in treatment protocols was resisted by many traditional practitioners at the time precisely because the causal story wasn't clear. But EBP adherents were often early adopters of the new treatment; what mattered was results, not complete understanding of the physiology.

4. *Externalized Authority*: In terms of authority structures, EBP locates authority outside the individual, in the body of knowledge that medical research and practice have developed over time. It advocates literature searches rather than relying solely on clinical judgment. It advocates questioning traditional practices rather than submitting to the authority of practitioners who embody that tradition. It advocates developing decision-making rubrics, and so downplays the importance of learning to model an expert doctor/teacher.

This aspect of EBP has proved to be a major barrier to its implementation in practice. Medicine has a very hierarchical structure, and any challenges to that structure, whether an earlier patient right's movement, or the team approach to medical decision-making, have proven difficult to implement. Because EBP incorporates a structure that allows for a lowly resident to challenge a senior attending if she or he has read the relevant studies, its full implementation would represent a distinct shift in the culture of medicine, one that has certainly not yet taken place (Timmermans and Berg, 2003, p. 160).

Summary of Differences

At this level of abstraction, clinical judgment and EBP provide two very different pictures of how medical care should be structured. In the clinical judgment model, we see something closely akin to the guild system, with experienced practitioners playing the role of guild master, and residents as apprentices being inducted into the practice by hands-on learning designed to shape their hands and minds in almost unconscious ways. In its emphasis on medicine as art, and focus on particularities, clinical judgment fits a model of Aristotelian practical wisdom in many ways. EBP, in contrast, offers a disenchanted medical practice, stripped of the mysterious knowledge and power of the individual practitioner. On this model, knowledge is available to anyone with good research skills. Diagnosis and treatment can be codified in decision-trees, and the standards of good practice are no longer set by individual practitioners. Instead, best practices are determined by large-scale studies and imposed on practitioners, whether they want them or not. While it is certainly true that in practice the difference between these two models is blurred, they nonetheless offer very different paradigms of medical care. In the next section, I turn to the question of how a shift as fundamental as this one affects the way that care is provided, how it affects caregivers themselves in their development as caregivers, and, finally, how the strengths and weaknesses of both models might be addressed.

Knowledge and Care

In many ways, the switch from clinical judgment to EBP has been a positive move for providing medical care. The most basic impetus behind moving to EBP is a concern to identify treatments that are the most effective, and then implement them. Almost no one would argue against this goal, and it represents the most significant aspect of the success of EBP. Implemented properly, EBP generates a higher standard of care for patients, and for that reason alone, it has been almost unchallenged in its takeover of medicine.

A second reason for the success of EBP is that it corrects one of the long-standing weaknesses in medical practice. Because the clinical judgment model of training is so heavily practice oriented, it can prevent the accumulation of new knowledge or updated practices. In their residency, students are shown the right way to do something, and then they practice doing that same technique over and over until they can do it the same way every time. This is a very effective way to teach techniques if you want people to always do the same thing, and to do it in the same way every time. Studies have shown that once a doctor has been trained, she or he will probably keep doing the same techniques for the rest of her life. Even though doctors are required to take continuing education classes throughout the rest of their careers, social scientists who study medicine note that very few doctors change the way they do things as a result of these classes—they keep on doing what they were trained to do when they were a student. Physicians, of course, are hardly the only people susceptible to this dynamic. Under the rubric of 'behavioral lock-in,' it is a phenomena of interest to sociologists, economists, and the like (Barnes et al., 2004).

To counter this, EBP requires continual revisiting of the literature, to find out what practices are regarded as best practices, and why. This demotion of practice-based settled wisdom in favor of continual investigation into new research has the potential to train doctors to think in terms of regularly revising techniques, rather than doing the same thing over and over. It is not surprising, of course, that this is a great strength of EBP, since it is precisely what EBP is designed to do—to keep medical caregivers engaged in an ongoing process of learning about and implementing best practices, rather than being trained at one period and then doing what one has been trained to do for the rest of one's career.

EBP also has the potential to diminish the hierarchical nature of medical practice and training by establishing an exterior authority to which all parties are subject. On the traditional clinical judgment model, authority is located in seniority (which roughly correlates with experience), so that the more senior a physician is, the harder it is to challenge anything she or he says. On an EBP model, on the other hand, even a resident can raise questions or challenges based on literature reviews. Studies have demonstrated that while EBP has not radically changed the authority structure of medical education, it has increased the incidence of residents who find ways to work around senior colleagues whose judgment is problematic—that is, the advent of EBP has increased the number of residents who will search out alternative views, find second opinions from other senior staff, and the like based on the knowledge they have found via research (Timmermans and Berg, 2003).

So, EBP has not gotten rid of the hierarchical nature of medical education, but it has diminished it to some degree—and from the perspective of an ethics of care, this is (all things being equal) a positive shift. Autocratic hierarchies (and what powerful hierarchy does not become autocratic to some degree?) generate problematic systemic behaviors in those who work within them, they diminish the focus on patient care and substitute maintenance of authority as the ultimate value, and present various other pathologies. To the extent that caregivers can function within more of a team structure and less of a benevolent despot structure, they function better in terms of providing patient care (Wagner, 2000).

So far, I have written largely about physicians and their training, but medical care, especially acute care, is not just provided by physicians. There is a wide range of caregivers in any health care system, from therapists to technologists to nurses. Nurses are particularly central to medical care because they provide the bulk of actual care in most acute care settings. Nursing was originally developed as a subsidiary practice, one that required nurses to submit to physician's authority and to care for their patients' well-being. This generated a serious tension for nurses when a physician's directives were not in a patient's best interest. As nursing has developed as a profession, one which now defines itself independently of physician control, nurses have increasingly argued that they bring a distinct perspective to patient care, and should be considered authorities in fields that represent their own areas of expertise.

In the context of the clinical judgment model, however, nursing's claim to an independent perspective on the good of the patient was challenging to substantiate, since clinical judgment was assumed to be the prerogative of a physician's judgment—nurses were not generally included as experts in clinical assessment, at least not in situations where their judgment conflicted with that of the treating physician. The hierarchical nature of the clinical judgment model worked to disempower nurses, and it is not surprising that nursing as a profession has welcomed the switch to EBP and considers it a timely and empowering move.

EBP has also been welcome because it establishes a way for nursing to provide evidence of the benefits of nursing practice. Skilled nursing care makes a huge and demonstrable difference in patient outcomes, but because medicine tends to be thought of in terms of what doctors do, cost-cutting often takes the form of cutting nurses, and replacing them with untrained aides. EBP has provided the means for nursing organizations to document the toll this takes on patient care, and to demonstrate that best practices require adequate provision of nursing care.

At the same time that the diminished hierarchical nature of EBP has empowered nursing, however, it has also generated, paradoxically, a potential problem. Nursing defines the care it gives in holistic terms, and emphasizes the need to provide care to a patient across all the various aspects of human life—physical, emotional, social, and spiritual. EBP, however, focuses on measurable data from large-scale studies. This data is valuable, but it can also screen out factors (emotional, social and spiritual) that are important for patients and for the nurses who care for them, but are not easily quantified or studied. This brings us to one of the potential weaknesses of EBP.

EBP operates with an ideal of medical knowledge that makes large-scale double-blind studies the 'gold standard' for medical knowledge (Timmermans and Berg, 2003). There are good reasons for this; large-scale studies avoid the problems of idiosyncratic results or non-representative samples that smaller studies produce, and double-blind studies minimize researchers' confirmation bias or worries about sponsorship affecting results. In terms of scientific adequacy, these criteria are perfectly sensible. But they also can serve to limit what counts as knowledge in ways that are problematic. To pick one example that has been widely discussed in the literature, pharmaceutical protocols are far easier to study and compare using wide-scale double-blind studies than are non-pharmaceutical techniques. Consider trying to do a study of the effectiveness of standard pain medications versus non-pharmaceutical techniques such as relaxation techniques, massage, and the like. Both providers and patients will know which treatment subjects get, so the comparison cannot be blind. One treatment involves interpersonal factors that the other does not (who performs the massage will likely make a difference, for example), and interpreting results will be difficult since one treatment modality involves so many complicating factors while the other involves a simple medication. Obviously, these differences are not insurmountable, and the proponents of EBP recognize the range of research that can be useful in evaluating treatment (Howick, 2011), but the fact remains that it is simply easier to provide evidence for some types of treatment than for others.

Because of the nature of the two protocols, the one will easily and relatively quickly yield lots of evidence; the other is less likely to be studied, and will have difficulty finding funding if a researcher does decide to pursue it. (Large pharmaceutical companies, not surprisingly, prefer to fund studies of pharmaceuticals.) When one does a literature review, then, looking for techniques of pain management, what one will find are extensive studies of various pharmaceutical therapies, and perhaps some mention of alternative treatments. Best practices will almost automatically lean toward the use of pharmaceuticals. They have been studied extensively and the evidence on them is of high quality, while alternative treatments have far less in the way of supporting evidence, fewer studies on smaller populations, and problems of limited sample sizes and researcher personal involvement.

Because many of the techniques that nursing offers in terms of concrete patient care are aimed at the holistic good of the patient, then, nursing care offers a range of practices that fall outside the boundary of the paradigm cases for which evidence can be easily obtained. This doesn't mean that nursing care doesn't offer important support for patients. It means, rather, that EBP provides a model that focuses the field of study on a limited range of evidence. But those limitations affect different medical specializations in different ways, and it does put nursing at a disadvantage in terms of demonstrating the nurse's value and expertise in the medical context.

Nurses are not the only medical professionals critical of EBP for its tendency to encourage narrow, formulaic reasoning in medicine. Physicians have been extremely critical as well, and have noted that the sometimes simplistic account of evidence, coupled with rigid decision-making procedures, results in care that is anything but patient-centered. More than this, the care guidelines derived from studies of patients with no co-morbidities may map very poorly onto patient care for the complex cases physicians actually face in real practice (Greenhalgh et al., 2014). Good clinical judgment skills remain important for good medical care, and EBP alone is not a substitute for such skills.

The change in hierarchical structure, then, has both positive and negative potential. On the one hand, it offers room for a more democratic, less top-down authority structure; on the other, it may also screen out or diminish the potential for finding therapies that are outside the pharmaceutical paradigm within which it works.

The two different results occur because what EBP substitutes for the old hierarchy—seniority/experience—is replaced by statistical studies. This still represents a hierarchy of sorts, though one that is based on type of knowledge rather than the person knowing. Any system of knowledge, of course, must incorporate some sort of hierarchy, since knowledge inherently is defined in contrast to lesser epistemic states (beliefs, mere opinions, ungrounded guesses), and there is nothing untoward about the sheer fact of that hierarchy. But any hierarchical ranking will (perhaps necessarily) also generate particular blind spots.

As it happens, it also seems to me that EBP is better situated to guard against blind spots insofar as it has undergone extensive review of what its own criteria may omit (Thorne, 2016) and also insofar as it remains continually open to challenges based on good data (Wajman et al., 2018). While it may not be the case that some treatment protocols can generate the same type of data as pharmaceutical studies, they can, nonetheless, demonstrate that in terms of outcome they may (or may not, depending on the protocol) be among the contenders for 'best practices' status. So, in the same way that EBP has the potential for diminishing authority hierarchies in medical practice, it also has the potential to allow for evidentiary support for alternative therapies, so long as those evaluating the evidence do not make features such as 'double-blind' a screen to exclude such protocols.

This brings us to yet another significant issue in the switch from clinical judgment to EBP; namely, the focus on outcomes. The dominant paradigm in medicine for centuries has been based on understanding the mechanisms of how treatments work—in many ways this was the fundamental basis for physician's claims to be the ultimate authority in medicine. In the early years of Western medicine, the mechanisms invoked were relatively dubious, and based on highly questionable accounts of physiology. One has only to read early discussions of the mechanisms whereby treatments such as bleeding and the administration of purgatives were justified to see, with the wisdom of hindsight, that past claims to expertise were based on dubious physiological reasoning indeed. But as the science of human physiology has improved, so have the explanations, and many protocols are well designed to work with what we know about the human organism to achieve positive results.

So, the switch to an outcomes-based model demanded by EBP has been one of the most aspects of EBP that has generated the greatest resistance. And it is easy to see why—an emphasis on physiological knowledge is clearly relevant to thinking about possible treatments, and understanding how a disease affects the various organ systems can lead to better treatment. But in some cases, treatments that are very effective have been rejected by doctors because they don't understand how that treatment could work. A good example of this in Western medicine is acupuncture. Most Western doctors will not use acupuncture, even though it has been shown to be effective for the treatment of a number of illnesses. The reason they won't use it is that they can't figure out how it works—they can't understand the physiological mechanisms involved—and so they assume that it is not real medicine.

On an EBP model, the central question is not whether we know how it works, but whether it works, and there is considerable data that acupuncture can be effective in certain cases for certain types of relief. So long as this can be well substantiated, then, an EBP model would advocate using acupuncture where it has been shown to be effective (keeping in mind that a therapy of this sort will be subject to the same sorts of difficulties in terms of research as the pain control therapies mentioned earlier: one simply cannot do a double-blind study wherein patients and researchers don't know who is and who isn't getting acupuncture, for obvious reasons.)

From an ethics of care perspective, EBP has the potential to inculcate epistemic humility in medical practitioners in ways that could be positive.

Because EBP builds into the practice of medicine the recognition that practitioners do not always understand exactly how or why things work, but can still recognize when they work, it encourages an openness to new techniques, and to changes in treatments that make practitioners less a source of absolute knowledge. This could shift the authority structures of medical practice in ways that are healthy. There is a tendency, less today than in decades past, but still occasionally on view, for physicians to think of themselves as standing in a place closely approximating God. This exalted status was natural enough: physicians often do control access to the treatment or surgery needed to stave off death or disfigurement, their knowledge is arcane and beyond the understanding of most lay people, and they speak in a language that is foreign to many of us, work in a strange temple with miraculous machines, and so on. And like any group that has the legal right, under certain conditions, to demand obedience (airline pilots sometimes confuse themselves with God for the same reason), physicians and the laity alike tend to assume that they are a breed apart.

But the attitude encouraged by EBP encourages a more realistic (and perhaps more humane) understanding of medical knowledge. Rather than an absolute gap between practitioners and patients, EBP builds in the recognition that any single practitioner will be limited in knowledge, that patients who are engaged in their own treatment may have insights to offer, and that a team approach to decision-making is generally a better technique than top-down autocracy. Epistemic humility is a better basis for a caregiver/patient relationship, it leads to better care overall, and it is a healthy trait for a caregiver to cultivate.

To see why this might be so, we need only think about what goes on when patient and physician are in the process of trying to diagnose a condition and consider treatments. When patient and physician alike recognize that the physician is not omniscient, the patient is freer to question and challenge claims that the physicians makes. She or he is also more likely to report back when a treatment seems not to be working (Groopman, 2007). Both of these lead to better patient outcomes overall. Further, when the physician is seen as a knowledgeable, but limited, human being, patients are more willing to recognize mistakes as mistakes, rather than respond to honest errors with lawsuits (Kachalia et al., 2010).

In terms of professional relations, likewise, epistemic humility is an important virtue to develop. Physicians who recognize their own limitations are more likely to recognize and be grateful for the alternative perspectives and specialized knowledge of other professionals, particularly nurses. Nurses in an acute care setting see patients over much more extended periods of time, they are often present for the interactions between family and patient, and their insight is invaluable in many cases in understanding why a patient who has been doing well suddenly seems to be needing more pain medication, or is suddenly much less compliant. Social workers and chaplains, too, can add to the care team's understanding of just what is going on in any given case.

But one loses access to this vital information if one is convinced of one's own epistemic authority. Absolute confidence in one's own knowledge is not a good attitude from which to learn from others.

In a number of ways, then, an ethics of care can find good reasons for evaluating the switch to EBP as largely positive. EBP can lessen problematic hierarchies in medicine, open up the range of professionals who can legitimately contribute to medical knowledge, and build in mechanisms for continual improvements of care. It holds practitioners to higher standards than is sometimes the case with the clinical judgment model, and makes standards of care explicit and based on clear evidence.

But the switch to EBP is not without its critics, and their concerns also need to be considered. The most widely discussed concern about EBP has been its privileging of large-scale statistical studies and meta-analysis over experience and the trained clinical judgment that develops over years of practice. Many within the practice of medicine have raised this issue (Groopman, 2007; Buetow and Kenealy, 2000), others have defended EBP against these charges (Parker, 2005), and it is clearly an issue that resonates with many practitioners. From the perspective of an ethics of care, how should this concern be evaluated?

Care theorists have emphasized the importance of particularized knowledge and a focus on concrete cases for care. Noddings, for example, argues that traditional ethical theorizing is flawed precisely because it focuses on abstract universal principles, often at the expense of the vulnerable or powerless (Noddings, 1989, p. 43). Caring for another, especially when that other is very vulnerable, requires sensitivity to individual aspects of that other's life and person in ways that are undermined, many care theorists argue, by a reliance on abstract principles. Care ethics analyses of the moral status of abortion, for example, generally reject any simplified absolute principles. The particularities of various individuals, situations, and contexts make any single, principle-based analysis too simplistic to be adequate for the complexities of human lives (Noddings, 1984; Sevenhuisjen, 2004; Held, 2006; Slote, 2007). From the perspective of an ethics of care, any attempt to resolve the issue with a simplistic principle will fail to provide an adequately caring response.

This perspective on ethical reasoning can be extended to the context of medical diagnosis and treatment. Abstract accounts of how any condition should be treated, or over-reliance on statistical reasoning in the absence of recognizing individual variation and particularity, can be the opposite of good care. Attending to particularity is a requirement of care, both ethically and medically. It can be much easier to accommodate a focus on particularity in the context of clinical judgment than on an EBP model. One of the common criticisms of EBP practice, for example, is that because it relies so heavily on data derived from large-scale studies, and because large-scale studies usually exclude participants with multiple (and confounding) conditions, the treatment protocols it mandates do not always fit well for specific patients with complicated conditions. Treatment protocols tested on relatively healthy middle-aged patients, for example, may not be optimal for elderly patients with multiple health problems, poor diets, and little mobility.

I have already mentioned earlier that EBP is also problematic because of the way that it privileges certain treatment modalities and downplays others. Again, from the perspective of an ethics of care, the specifics of this issue are problematic. Medical care is given in an increasingly technological, mechanized environment. Contemporary reimbursement structures are set up to reimburse caregivers for interventions, but rarely for their time or attention. Much of contemporary medicine emphasizes, in Daniel Callahan's phrase, cure rather than care, often to the detriment of the quality of life of those cared for (Callahan, 1992). To the extent that EBP contributes to this dynamic, it is problematic.

In terms of how care is provided, EPB also offers another set of potential problems having to do with rationing. Health care costs in the Western world are astronomically high. The US spent 17.7% of its GDP on health care in 2013, roughly $9,086 per person. This is almost 50% more than the next highest spender (in terms of percentage of GDP) and almost double what the U.K. spends per person (Squires and Anderson, 2015). This sort of spending is not something that any country can afford, and so most Western countries are trying to find methods of cutting back on expenses. Generally, this takes the form of rationing: deciding that only some people will get certain treatments, and others won't.

One of the most common forms of rationing occurs when an insurance company decides that it will only pay for particular treatments. There may be three different medicines that can treat high blood pressure, for example, but the company will only pay for one of them, usually the cheapest. But if the insurance company announced that it only wants to pay for the cheapest medicines, the people who pay for that insurance would complain, and the company might lose business.

In response, many insurance companies (and in countries like England that have state-provided medical care, some government organizations) have started producing what are called 'care guidelines.' The guidelines tell doctors what medicines they can prescribe for what conditions, how many days of hospitalization they can prescribe for particular cases, and the like. The basis for the guidelines is supposed to be the sort of evidence we've seen advocated by EBP. But cost-effectiveness is among the criteria used for determining these guidelines. In itself, this is not necessarily unacceptable. The notion of something being 'cost-effective' should mean that the treatment provides more benefit for its cost than any other alternative treatment. This can be a valid consideration. If, for example, sinus infections can be treated almost as effectively by salt water flushing as by antibiotics, then it might make sense to use salt water (which is almost free) rather than an expensive antibiotic. So, most studies of medicines and treatments now include an examination of the cost of the treatment and its relationship to expected benefit.

There are two problems, however, with the inclusion of cost-effectiveness in the analysis of treatments. One problem is that it mixes categories of evidence. The second is that insurers have a very strong bias in favor of keeping costs down, and this bias makes suspect their ability to fairly weigh costs against other considerations. These two problems work in tandem. A scientific study can often provide good evidence that a treatment is effective against a particular condition and can compare the treatment to other comparable treatments. But when we start analyzing economics along with clinical effectiveness, the scientific objectivity of the researchers is called into question. Worse than this, the weighting of scientific and health factors against economic considerations is always subjective.

Imagine that a particular medication is moderately effective—it works part of the time, but doesn't work in many cases. In addition, it has serious side effects—people who take it feel sick and nauseous much of the time, and it is harmful to a person's liver. Another medication is more effective, and does not have these side effects. But now imagine, as well, that the manufacturing processes of these two medicines make the second one cost ten times what the first one does. How should a researcher weight that cost difference against the effectiveness of the medicine? Most people would rather take the second medicine, of course, but there aren't any objective criteria available to us that tells us at what point the medical effectiveness and lack of side effects outweigh cost differences. When a third-party payer is in charge of weighing these factors, side effects and decreased effectiveness can seem trivial compared to the potential for saving money.

EBP is supposed to increase people's quality of care by identifying the treatments that have the best outcomes. But when cost becomes part of the evaluation of outcomes, however, the 'best' outcome may be the best outcomes from an accounting perspective, rather than the perspective of the patient. One of the tensions that EBP cannot resolve simply by looking for yet more evidence is the question of what sorts of things are to count as 'best' when researchers evaluate best practices.

Of course, the clinical judgment model cannot resolve this issue, either. But in the case of clinical judgment, the problem is less acute because that picture of medical knowledge is less dependent on an evidential model that privileges statistical decision-making. Reliance on the clinician's judgment allows more room for individualizing such decisions, rather than making them on the basis of generalities and cost/benefit analyses.

One final issue is worth noting in terms of some of the weaknesses of EBP. EBP incorporates a notion of best practices, and endorses a model of standardized care based on that concept. In many ways, this is a very positive change in medicine, as I noted earlier, because it encourages physicians using sub-standard or outdated treatment protocols to bring their treatments in line with an improved standard of care. Statistically, this has been shown to generate improvements in the standard of care and in patient health outcomes. But this improvement comes at a cost. Standardization raises the level of care being given in the worst cases, but it also can diminish the care given by the best practitioners. A skilled and experienced practitioner can often move more quickly to diagnosis than 'best practices' might dictate. Standardization of care will require the physician to make patients undergo possibly unnecessary tests and delays of treatment because that is the standard of care. Any system of standardization tends to have this effect: it improves the situation overall by bringing the lowest functioning professionals up to a common standard, but also diminishes the performance of the best professionals by requiring them to conform to a standard that may be lower than what they could otherwise provide.

Why Not Both? Medicine as Art and Science

Some people have argued that medicine should not see these two models as opposed to each other, but should instead try to adapt systems that incorporate the best aspects of both models (Karthikeyan and Pais, 2009). On this view, medical training would still involve lots of practice, learning hands-on treatment, and observing senior doctors who are good at clinical judgment, but this practical training would also include learning to do literature searches to obtain the most recent statistical studies, learning to check clinical judgment by quickly examining the decision-making rubrics, and the like.

But as in so many areas of life, this ideal is easier to imagine in the abstract than it is to implement in the real world. The problem is that the two models of medicine operate with such different conception of knowledge that each tends to undercut implementation of the other. One conception works with a picture of knowledge that has deep roots in the Aristotelian tradition, emphasizing the way that practical wisdom is gained by experience and habituation. The other conception operates with a more mathematical, computer-based account of rationality, focuses on data and statistics, and emphasizes abstraction rather than focusing on particularity. The more emphasis is placed on developing thinkers who exemplify one or the other type of rationality, the harder it will be to synthesize the two in ways that preserve the strengths of both.

There is no simple answer to this debate. On the one hand, the use of computerized decision processes can increase both speed and accuracy of diagnosis. For the better students, it can also generate a sensitivity to the symptoms they elicit from patients when taking a history, and train them in their basic understanding of standard diagnosis. On the other hand, computer-based diagnosis and reasoning can prevent doctors, young and old, from thinking outside the box, or exploring possibilities that are lower in the probability scale, but need to be considered nonetheless. After all, that a condition has a lower probability still entails that there is some probability that it does pertain. In terms of proposing treatments, likewise, over-reliance on decision-making protocols standardizes treatments, it is true, but that has both positive and negative effects. It can raise the lower levels of treatment for all patients, because it rules out out-moded or ineffective treatments. In so doing, it raises the standard of care for those who would have suffered from less-than-adequate treatments. But while it raises the lower half of the care spectrum, it also poses the risk of lowering the upper half—of lowering the truly superior care down to the level of accepted protocols.

In a similar way, both accounts of knowledge tend to generate blind spots in practitioners, but in different areas. EBP's picture of what counts as evidence, for example, encourages practitioners to preferentially choose certain types of treatments and ignore others. In a surprisingly wide variety of cases, the evidence that EBP relies on is not available, and in a small but important subset of those cases, the evidence cannot be made available, because the testing needed to generate truly adequate results from a scientific point of view would require subjecting patients to an unacceptable level of risk.

One of the solutions to this problem that EBP adopts is to establish different levels of evidence, so that the best evidence consists of widely duplicated, double-blind studies, either performed on large enough populations to be statistically reliable or generated by meta analyses. Other types of evidence are ranked, relative to this 'gold standard' in terms of reliability, from small-scale studies that either haven't been duplicated or weren't double-blind, to widespread observations from practitioners. This helps with the problem to some extent, since it acknowledges that there can be evidence that doesn't fit the scientific model exactly, but it doesn't resolve it entirely.

The problem is that while practitioners can know, intellectually, that the absence of evidence does not justify claims of inefficacy for a given treatment, in practice, the search for evidence does lead a practitioner to expect that evidence will accompany good treatment protocols, and will also lead him or her to be automatically biased toward treatment protocols that are based on large-scale studies. It is one thing to know intellectually that X could be a good treatment; it is quite another (especially in a litigious society such as the US) to set aside the lack of evidence and choose X when Y does offer evidence-based support. And, as we noted earlier, certain types of protocols lend themselves well to being tested (pharmaceutical treatments, especially, but also many surgical protocols), while others, especially ones that rely on time-intensive interaction with another person, don't lend themselves well to producing the sort of evidence that practitioners are trained to look for.

I will return to this point in a subsequent chapter, as I think it is part of a whole structural package that pushes modern medical practice toward ever-greater use of technology without much evaluation of whether that technology really gets us where we should be going. But that is an argument for another chapter; for this one, I am concerned with the way that EBP shapes patterns of thinking so that practitioners develop automatic preferences for treatments of certain sort, while just as automatically screening out alternative therapies that may be similar in effectiveness, but less demonstrably so due to the very type of therapy they offer.

There are ways of working around the blind spots that EBP can generate in practitioners, and it is certainly not the case that clinical judgment is free from blind spots. Those blind spots have been well documented in the sociological literature on medicine: the tendency of physicians, due to confirmation bias, to overestimate the positive benefits of procedures they have used in the past, underestimate the benefits of unfamiliar treatments; over-reliance on individual cases that are particularly memorable, rather than on statistical data, and the like. These are, in fact, the blind spots that EBP is designed to overcome, and it does that well. But in overcoming one set of blind spots, we usually set ourselves up with a whole other set of blinders, and that is the situation in which EBP can find itself today.

From the perspective of an ethics of care, there are reasons to be hesitant about the wholesale adoption of EBP. It has the potential to shape medical practitioners' thinking in ways that may make caregiving particularly difficult, given its tendency to privilege abstract statistical thinking over attention to the particularities of an individual patient. But to assume that this should result in care theorists rejecting EBP would be too simple. It offers a picture of what medical knowledge is, and how it functions that can improve care tremendously, and can validate the knowledge claims of individuals and groups who have traditionally been treated as less authoritative, and this is an important corrective for medical culture.

Ultimately, the question of how EBP is implemented, and the ways in which medical education and practice continue to incorporate some of the best aspects of the clinical judgment model will depend, in part, on other aspects of medical practice. As the cost of medicine continues to grow far faster than almost any other sector of the economy, pressure to economize will push health care systems to implement EBP in relatively simplistic and cost-effective ways. Resisting some of this pressure will require theorists and practitioners alike to articulate the value of skills and techniques made invisible by EBP, especially the values of interpersonal, caring relationships between caregivers and patients. It may be possible to demonstrate in some cases that there is evidence that time spent listening to patients, for example, offers a cost-effective way of delivering patient care. In other cases, where cost-effectiveness should not be the central goal of specific medical practices, it will be necessary to articulate the values that should structure the delivery of health care. For end of life care, for example, while it seems obviously important to keep costs reasonable, cost-effectiveness should not be the only goal that drives our reasoning.

The questions of how we frame the ends of medicine, and how that shapes the practice of caring in the context of the contemporary health care arena, are ones I will return to in the last chapter of this study. At this point, I want to note that one central issue that can be obscured by the knowledge claims generated by EBP is that there are questions to which EBP has no answers—and in some cases, these are the most important. As with any model of what counts as knowledge, however, EBP can create blind spots at the places where the knowledge it can generate runs up against its own limits. Unless we can articulate where it stops as an account of knowledge, and recognize that there are truths outside its ken, we will run into problems with the way it structures care, and with the way it shapes caregivers' character and care provision.

Notes

1 Much of the literature refers to evidence-based medicine (EBM), but because I use the term to refer to the practices of both physicians and nurses, evidence-based practice is more inclusive.

2 One area where the clinical judgment model still persists, and generates some interesting ethical conflicts in medical practice, is the area of research. Medical research warrants extensive moral scrutiny precisely because it focuses on obtaining evidence rather than on the good of the patient. Physicians implicitly or explicitly promise their patients that their central focus will be the patient's own best interests, an obligation generally referred to as the therapeutic obligation. Researchers are primarily focused on producing accurate results, and that sometimes requires putting patients at risk. Rules requiring research to undergo review by an institutional review board (IRB) and be subject to extensive reporting requirements reflect the potential for abuse, as do the safeguards designed to protect patients who think they are getting medical treatment from being misled into instead becoming unwitting experimental subjects. While good research is compatible with focusing on the best interests of a patient (Marquis, 1999), the two can also diverge in problematic ways.

3 Public Health and Free Markets

In the previous chapter, we saw some of the ways that contemporary health care has changed as the structure of knowledge in medicine has shifted from clinical judgment to evidence-based knowledge. These changes, of course, do not occur in a vacuum. They are accompanied by unprecedented changes in the technological tools available to health care workers, and accompanying economic changes. Economic forces form the focus of this chapter, which will examine the way economic considerations structure the delivery of care, and also the very nature of care itself. As part of that discussion, it will consider how that economic factors affect caregivers in terms of how they perform their role, and what sorts of people they become.

Economic issues in health care have become particularly fraught in the US in recent years, with politicized battles over 'death panels,' 'socialized medicine,' passage and attempted repeal of the Affordable Care Act, and continuing questions about Medicare and Medicaid budgets. While I cannot avoid all of these political debates, they are not the main focus of this chapter. Instead, what I will analyze are the ways that various economic structures affect the provision of care. That, it seems to me, is a valuable project regardless of where one stands on particular political issues. Information about how the free market functions to make care available or unavailable, how government subsidized health care serves the same purposes, and how systems of this sort impact caregivers themselves, it seems to me, is worthwhile, regardless of where one stands on various political questions.

The range of economic systems that can be used to provide health care is wide, from systems that rely completely on out-of-pocket payment by patients for any and all treatments; to systems involving third-party payers, whether insurance companies or government institutions; to national health systems that provide care to all citizens much on the model of public education in the US; to mixed-systems that patch together some features of all of these. In the space of one chapter, it is not possible to resolve all of the issues that can be generated by the patchwork of economic systems found in the world today; for the purposes of this chapter, I will think through the potential problems and positives of a spectrum of possible systems, beginning with an extreme free market model and working through to a completely publicly funded model. While I won't be specifically examining any of the existent systems, they will be used to offer guidance on how these systems do actually function in the real world, and how they have resolved some of the challenges each faces at a theoretical level. So, much as I did in the chapter on knowledge, I will start by describing relatively pure forms of the various economic possibilities, and the positives and negatives associated with each for providing care and for shaping caregiver/patient relationships in healthy ways.

The models to be examined here represent a spectrum of economic models about which economists have been arguing for decades. Should markets be completely unregulated, so that the invisible hand will generate the greatest benefit overall? Or are unregulated markets simply destined to implode and generate hugely expensive bubbles that destroy economic well-being for lengthy periods of time? Are free markets inherently destructive for the working classes, because they set up an inevitable clash between the owners of the means of production and the laborers? And so on. I will not resolve these debates. My interest here is far more narrow: how do these various models of economic structure affect the delivery of care, both in terms of what they intentionally provide (or do not provide) and in terms of what they produce as unintended side effects? How do they affect caregivers, and more specifically, how do they shape the character of those who provide health care within the various economic systems?

Free Market Systems

On one extreme end of the spectrum of possibilities, we find a model that maximizes the freedom of the market. On such a model, medical care is considered to be like any other commodity, and caregivers should be allowed to set their rates at whatever level the market will allow. Consumers will presumably make decisions about what they can afford as far as health care goes, and allocate funds accordingly, thus making the market as efficient (in the economic sense) as possible.[1]

In order for any market to perform efficiently, many economists assume, consumers need to be the ones who decide what they are willing to pay for. In the case of health care, then, individuals should be the ones to decide what treatments they are willing to pay for, and how much they are willing to pay, and they also need the freedom (and adequate sources of information) to choose the caregivers they think can offer the best ratio of affordability and competency. But in the contemporary world, consumers generally have no idea what various treatments cost, and have no way of ranking effectiveness of various practitioners, or any of the information necessary to make informed decisions.[2] Rather unrealistically, many libertarians nonetheless simply assume that those needing treatments or pharmaceuticals will have access to accurate information about side effects, possible dangers, and the like. In the absence of a government organization like the Food and Drug

Administration (FDA) that is tasked with providing consumers with relatively accurate information about pharmaceuticals, such an assumption is little more than magical thinking. Even theorists sympathetic to libertarianism have argued that basic concerns about information asymmetries, externalities and the reasonableness of certain types of paternalistic interventions make a purely libertarian system of regulating drugs and pharmaceuticals unworkable (Leland, 1979; Polsby, 1998); the situation only gets worse when the entire spectrum of medical treatments is considered.

I will set worries about adequate information in a true free market system aside, however, not because they are not important, but because they are both obvious and because there are so very many other reasons why a free market in medicine is an unworkable system. To see these other problematic aspects of a completely free market in medicine, we'll need to imagine a setting where people have absolute freedom to make their own health care choices, where medical care is available to all in just the same way that standard consumer goods are, and those who can pay for it can purchase whatever they think is best.

One major change in current medical practice that would need to accompany this free market is the removal of licensing requirements for professionals. Libertarians have argued that this is a necessity so that the supply side of medical care can operate on free market principles (Friedman, 1962; Baron, 1983). Professional guilds can certainly require certain levels of training for care providers who want to use particular titles, of course, so the American Medical Association might still have a monopoly on the use of the title of 'physician.' But in a true free market, the state cannot criminalize other providers who want to offer medical treatments of various sorts. If one's local barber wants to offer surgery as a sideline to his shaving business, for example, that should be a matter between him and anyone willing to pay for his services.

What one would find, on this model, is a large array of providers and treatments, running the gamut from totally bogus to highly qualified. Consumers would have to make their way through the system as best they could, paying for whatever they could out of pocket. The majority of what we think of as standard medicine today (MRIs and CT scans, open-heart surgery and lengthy courses of chemotherapy for cancer) would be far too expensive for most consumers, and so might be available for the very wealthy, if there was sufficient demand to keep them in existence at all. But for the average citizen, standard courses of treatment would be completely out of reach. One cannot pay for a $250,000 surgery on a yearly salary of $50,000, for example, so most major surgeries and prolonged treatment regimens would be inaccessible for the majority of the population. Most people, most of the time, would choose caregivers with far lower levels of training, and far less-effective treatments, for the simple reason that this is what they could afford.

It is clear, just thinking about this most basic free market system of health care, that much of the care provided would be markedly inferior to what almost anyone would consider adequate health care today. It would resemble something much closer to what one finds in many countries in the Global South, where resources are extremely scarce and the most vulnerable members of society (the poor, the old, the young) are largely without recourse in gaining access to even basic aspects of medical care. This highlights one of the challenges of thinking about medical care in the contemporary world, economically.

Health care is a tremendously expensive business, and it is likely to get more expensive in the future, not less, for a number of reasons, some of them having to do with the role that technology plays in health care. Unlike many other fields of business, where costs decrease as the field develops, health care is a field where costs increase as medicine becomes more successful at doing what it does. There are several reasons for this. One is that success in health care results in people living longer, and the longer someone lives, the more health care they will use, statistically speaking (Breyer and Felder, 2006). There are economic debates about how much longevity increases expenditures, and several economic studies have noted that the increase are often overestimated (Shang and Goldman, 2007; Werblow et al., 2007), but it remains the case that the better the system becomes at keeping people alive, the more expensive health care will become in turn.[3] Think, for example of the woman who survives her first heart attack and lives for another 20 years. She will, as a result of living 20 years longer, require significantly more health care dollars (to treat her ulcer, or her breast cancer, or her next heart attack) during the course of those 20 years.

Second, successful treatment frequently involves continued treatment: we can now treat conditions such as high blood pressure and diabetes, but successful treatment involves continuing to provide treatment over long periods of time (unlike, say, curing a broken leg or a ruptured appendix, whereby the cure is the end of the necessary treatment). So being able to treat conditions often doesn't decrease costs, but instead increases them, and for increasingly long times as our understanding of medicine gets better (Jönsson, 2002). Add to these dynamics the fact that medical treatments have gotten technologically more complex, a trend that will continue, and continue to make medical care that much more expensive, and one sees why cost control in medicine is an extremely difficult issue. I will return to some of these issues from an alternative vantage point when I take up the issue of technology in the next chapter, but for now the question is how they affect the economic structures that allow for medical provision.

Market mechanisms in medicine are complicated, in part, because medical treatment is unlike many other goods. People who need acute care, either to continue living or to simply be able to function reasonably well and without pain, generally are willing to trade off almost any amount of money for the chance to return to normal functioning. This is not surprising—money is the sort of good that we value instrumentally, while life, the absence of pain, and functionality tend to be much more intrinsic goods; that is, we want these things for their own sake, not because they are necessary for some further goals. Most people won't generally trade expected economic benefits against immediate threats to life or functionality, for fairly obvious reasons. This is one of the features of the economics of health care that makes basic market mechanisms problematic; there often is no upper limit to what people will pay to get acute medical care—they'll bankrupt the family, sell all they own, and do whatever they can to get needed care. But for markets to function efficiently, the goods exchanged need to be fungible, not something consumers will purchase no matter what the price.

Paradoxically, preventive and basic health care needs generate the opposite problem for the free market, Preventive care is something people often neglect, even when that neglect can lead to serious problems later on. This is frequently a matter of denial; the hope is that if one doesn't think about health problems, they'll just go away. When it comes to preventive care, then, market mechanisms tend to under-value people's health, while for acute care, market mechanisms fail because almost no price is too high. This makes health care market a particularly bad fit for free market systems of delivery.

Insurance, of course, responds to these factors. When people need acute care, they frequently need it to save either life or functionality, they need it immediately (or within a short time period), and its costs will be overwhelming. But they also know that they won't all need this type of treatment, and that they can't reliably predict who will and who won't. Studies have suggested that about 10% of patients account for the majority of health care expenditures (Berk and Monheit, 2001), but who will be in that 10% is very hard to predict. So, in the early part of the last century, as medical treatments became both more effective and more expensive at the same time, it became common to move away from a fee-for-service system that was relatively close to a free market, and to move instead to a system that involved some form of collectively provided medical care. While the first versions of collectivized health care were often company doctors (often hired by mining and railroad corporations) and physicians hired by lodges and other collective groups, in the 1940s, with the rise of unions and collective bargaining, health care began, increasingly, to be provided by insurance (Starr, 1982).

Further, purchasing insurance also addresses the second factor, because insurance systems are frequently designed to encourage people to seek care before conditions become acute and expensive. Preventive care can be a win-win for both consumers and insurers when it prevents serious health problems because the consumers enjoy the benefits of remaining healthy, while the insurer enjoys the benefits of lower costs. In the next section of this chapter, we'll turn to questions of how insurance systems structure care, but before we turn to that, it is worth spending a few pages on the positives and negatives of an extreme free market system for the provision of care and for the providers who work in such a system.

There are, first, a number of clear and perhaps insurmountable negatives to a pure free market system when it comes to providing care. Access to what most in the contemporary world would consider adequate medical care would be unavailable to a large range of the population. What would take its place, presumably, is a wide range of people offering care of various sorts, from herbalists and faith healers to nurses and technicians, side by side with a variety of hucksters only too happy to prey on the vulnerability of those facing serious illness. Caregivers themselves would need to limit the care they could offer to those willing to pay, which would require that they demand proof of solvency in advance of treatment. This would be a barrier to developing caring relationships, obviously, since caregivers could not promise ongoing care in advance, nor could they provide care based on need rather than ability to pay.

This is a straightforward logical result of a free market system, which requires relationships to be economically mediated. Whether one thinks that making caregiver/patient relationships completely economically mediated is a good thing or a bad thing will depend, in part, on what one thinks the ultimate ends of medicine should be (Pellegrino, 1999). If one considers medical care to be one consumer good among many, then presumably one would also think that making medical relationships purely economic transactions would be unproblematic. If, on the other hand, one thinks that medical care is among the goods that should not be turned into a complete commodity, then the specter of turning caregiver/patient relationships into a matter of pure economic transaction is deeply troubling. The final chapter of this book returns to the question of the ultimate ends of medicine; for present purposes, it is perhaps sufficient to note that medicine has never been understood to be a pure consumer good. While there are many aspects of medical care that can, plausibly, be distributed via basic market mechanisms, there are also major aspects of medical care that would go deeply wrong in a completely free market system.

One obvious aspect of health care that has not traditionally been considered appropriate for the free market is the caregiver/patient relationship. Physicians' relationships with patients have historically been understood, by both sides, as a fiduciary relationship; a relationship whereby the more vulnerable party can legitimately trust the professional to act in ways that are in the patient's best interests. But a free market relationship is not a fiduciary relationship since the provider acts out of profit motives, not out of concern for the other's best interests. At the very least, then, a pure free market system would drastically change basic medical relationships in ways that could be expected to be detrimental to the patient's well-being.

Further, and rather obviously, in a pure free market medical system, there would be no guarantee of care in emergency cases or whenever a person was unable to provide proof of capacity for payment. Unless one was already wealthy enough to cover any contingency, things like emergency rooms offering care to any who need it would disappear, as would other forms of guaranteed emergency care. Presumably, individuals could purchase various forms of coverage to ensure care in emergency situations, but without relatively heavy-handed government regulation, this coverage might or might not be reliable. In this and any number of other ways, a pure fee-for-service model would produce a system where the relationships between caregivers and patients has fundamentally changed.

Fee for service shapes the caregiver/patient relationship in any number of ways. For one thing, it can give a patient more power, since the caregiver is paid directly, and the patient can always take their business elsewhere if they are displeased. This, of course, is the power often pointed to in libertarian analyses. In other ways, however, given the often dire necessity that generates trips to a caregiver, it can give the caregiver an almost exploitive level of power vis-à-vis the patient. When patients are desperate, they are often willing to pay any price, even one that might bankrupt the entire family, to get treatment. They are also particularly vulnerable to exploitation and manipulation by unscrupulous service providers.

Further, when the caregiver has a direct financial interest in marketing a service, both diagnosis and treatment decisions can be affected detrimentally, even when the caregiver has good intentions. Health care workers, ideally, should not be in a situation where their financial interests run counter to the best interests of the patient. Studies repeatedly demonstrate, in fact, that financial incentives do affect physicians' clinical decisions (Hillman et al., 1989; Hemenway et al., 1990; Gruber and Owings, 1994; Mitchell, 2008). Recognizing this is clearly not to denigrate physicians' characters, but simply to note that they are human, like the rest of us. In fact, given standard economic assumptions about rational decision-making, it would be bizarre to expect that physicians would not be affected by financial concerns. But because health care is a practice that involves such deep vulnerabilities on the part of patients, proposing to make it a practice mediated entirely by the market produces a particularly dangerous situation for patients.

The various negatives of a completely free market in health care are obvious, and sufficient to make it obviously unacceptable from an ethics of care standpoint. But having noted this, it is also worth recognizing that there are some features of this system that are positives from the perspective of an ethics of care. First, note that this system does allow for a wide range of caregivers. Instead of funneling all medical care through the narrow gateway of physician supervision, this is a system that allows for a huge network of caregivers. And while many will be charlatans, many more will offer treatments that might, in some cases, serve the needs of those who get them, as well as the modern medical equivalent. A young mother suffering from post-partum depression might find that the herbalist down the street who spends extensive time talking about the loneliness of new motherhood, techniques for breastfeeding that don't hurt so much, and the need to get sleep whenever possible really does offer help; whether it is the herbs, or the advice, or the companionship (or all three) may not matter all that much. Likewise, being able to have a barber slice off that stupid wart while cutting one's hair might be a bit more cost-effective than having to make an appointment weeks in advance to let a clearly over-qualified physician do exactly the same thing.

For a large range of non-life threatening conditions, contemporary systems of health care offer what can only be considered overkill. Those performing procedures often have far more training than is strictly needed, the context within which treatments are offered is far more complex than necessary, and what many patients need (a listening ear, practical advice about basic life skills, simple and obvious procedures) is in increasingly short supply. Now, obviously, there are multiple treatments that do require the enormous complexity of the contemporary medical delivery system. I do not want to denigrate the truly wonderful things contemporary medicine can do. But caregivers themselves regularly lament the fact that they cannot give their patients time and attention; they regularly feel frustration about the way that simple conditions become medicalized beyond any degree of rationality, and so on.

What our thought experiment reminds us is that regulation, even the best-meant regulation, always has side effects. These side effects may or may not be worth the price, but unless we can name them, we cannot think of ways to mitigate them. The free market model of medicine, even with all of its potential drawbacks, does have the virtue of reminding us that protecting a sphere of freedom within which individuals can design their own systems of offering care, and within which others can seek out the care that meets their own perceived needs, can be valuable for both caregivers and care receivers. Recent moves within contemporary medicine to increase the range of caregivers (increasing the availability and freedom of midwives and nurse practitioners, for example) is a very small step in the direction of widening the scope of those who can provide care. It also allows us to begin to distinguish the sorts of care that various people can give, rather than requiring all care to be provided under the oversight of a physician. Likewise, the general trend of patients turning to a variety of sources of information on the internet al.so represents a broadening of our sense of where medical care can come from. Some of the sources, of course, are either professionally supported information sites or commercial sites, but some are simply forums where groups of people facing the same diagnosis come to discuss their symptoms, their treatments, and their opinions. In some cases, the level of disinformation is high, in others low, and the individual searching the web needs to be careful about what he or she accepts, but the presence of such groups has been tremendously helpful to many people.

As noted earlier, however, in spite of this positive aspect of a pure free market system, it is not a reasonable alternative for most in the contemporary world. Given that the costs of medical care can be catastrophic, but are somewhat unpredictable, it is to be expected that most medical care will be provided for either by some form of insurance or by public financing. And insurance itself can be either a matter of private choice or public regulation (or any number of complicated mixtures of the two). Insurance that functions as a market product is a smaller step away from a pure free market system than a regulated insurance market, so that will be the next step for our consideration along the spectrum of economic structures.

Market-Based Insurance Systems

For the market in insurance to resemble something like a free market, the current system in the US would have to be radically changed. The vast majority of insurance is currently provided through one's employer as part of a total employment package, it is an untaxed benefit, and other than minor marginal choices (preferred provider organizations [PPOs] vs. health maintenance organizations [HMOs]; the addition of a dental rider, etc.), consumers have little to no say in the choice of the insurance they carry. Things are different for the self-insured, obviously, but given the vagaries of the insurance market, the self-insured may have no choices at all if no carrier wants to cover them. Although the recent passage of the Affordable Care Act may change patterns of insurance in the US in the coming years, it seems unlikely that the US will move away from an employer-provider model of insurance. In order to examine how a market-based insurance system could affect care, it will be necessary to abstract from the present system in the US and consider an alternative.

Let us imagine, then, a system whereby insurance is not provided by employers, but is purchased by individuals, who have a reasonable range of plans and coverage from which to choose. This would be what Daniel Shapiro refers to as market health insurance, perhaps supplemented with tax credits or supplements for the indigent and for the uninsurable (Shapiro, 1998). Insurance carriers offer coverage for a specified range of conditions and treatments, and consumers select insurance on the basis of an optimal ratio between cost and coverage. Treatment for conditions not covered by insurance is available only on an out-of-pocket basis. A system whereby consumers made decisions about what insurance plans to purchase would allow market mechanisms to affect the health care system; presumably, consumers would want coverage for the conditions they would expect to foresee, though they might forego coverage for catastrophic or rare conditions. Premiums could reflect the level of co-payments or deductibles, and so on. A system somewhat like this currently obtains in Singapore, where citizens are required to contribute a pre-defined percentage of their wages to medical savings accounts, which they can then use to purchase insurance plans of their own choosing.

Clearly, such a system resolves at least some of the access problems of the pure free market system, since presumably such a system would allow a much larger number of patients to get higher level treatments than if they had to pay out of pocket. It would permit much greater continuity of care, and might address some of the problems of low-quality or ineffective treatments if insurance companies regulated providers to ensure a reasonable level of effectiveness. Access to insurance could also mitigate some of the more problematic issues that a fee-for-service system generates, since the presence of a third-party payer could shift the dynamics of the caregiver/ patient relationship. On the one hand, insurance can limit the power of the patient to choose caregivers, thus limiting customer freedom of choice (but also, in some cases, protecting the patient from charlatans). On the other hand, insurance can also limit the decisions caregivers can make by limiting the range of treatment options (covering only generic medications, for example) or by structuring reimbursements to encourage certain types of care over others. This can be a positive feature when it improves patient care, but is often experienced as a negative intrusion into the caregiver/ patient relationship by customers. The only unqualified benefit of insurance systems overall, it would seem, is an increase in access to health care.

That access would come at a cost, of course, since the added layer of complexity that the insurance market adds to the health care system increases costs for everyone, patients and caregivers alike. For 2016, the total revenues from premiums and administrative services for the five largest health insurers in the US totaled over $360 billion (Schoen and Collins, 2017), and similar revenues are noted for the years immediately prior. Other costs are more difficult to quantify, but administrative costs in the US are almost three times higher than they are in Canada, and some of those costs presumably are due to the complexities of dealing with insurance carriers (Woolhandler et al., 2003). Most physicians' offices in the US, for example, need to have one or more full-time employees who do nothing but deal with insurance companies. Health care systems as a whole likewise have extensive administrative expenses due to their interactions with insurance carriers. Recent studies indicate that the costs of handling insurance claims runs around 14.5% for primary care visits, 25% for emergency department visits, and 13% for ambulatory surgical procedures (Tseng et al., 2018). It is worth noting that these are the costs associated with the health network's handling costs. They do not include insurance premiums, charges, or other profits that accrue to the insurance company itself.

While $360 billion is, of course, a very large amount of money, this does not, by itself, show that too much money is spent on insurance, nor that insurance companies make too much in profits. Average reported profits for health insurance companies generally have remained somewhere between 5% and 7% of revenue for a number of years, and this is not an exceptionally high rate of profit, though it is a healthy one. Insurance companies report that they spend approximately 80% of premiums on actual medical expenses (Reinhardt, 2017). But it is the case that the added layers of bureaucracy, administrative costs, inefficiencies, patient time spent dealing with insurers, and all the other complications that the insurance market introduces into the health care market decreases overall efficiency. It is also worth noting that a significant proportion of health insurance premiums do not pay for health care, but rather for administrative costs. These added costs are part of what makes American health care so expensive. In countries that regulate insurance carriers more heavily (requiring specific levels of coverage, limiting premiums and profits, and so on), these costs are not so high.

Insurance systems (either publicly regulated or free market) also generate types of behavior that economists consider sub-optimal from the perspective of economic efficiency. The first is what economists call moral hazard—the creation of a greater level of risk-taking on the part of those covered by insurance. Closely related to moral hazard in the classical sense is a second issue that some commentators include under moral hazard: the tendency to over-utilize services due to the presence of a third-party payer. The first sort of moral hazard would be represented by people who are somewhat more motivated to skip taking their blood pressure medications because of their confidence that any health problems this generates will be covered by their insurance. An example of the second type would be physicians who order (and patients who undergo) tests that are unnecessary but covered by insurance.

Insurance companies can take a number of steps to mitigate these problems. Co-pays exist, in part, to encourage patients to limit tests and treatments. Some HMOs have experimented with paying physicians a flat fee per patient rather than reimbursement for each office visit and treatment. Many insurance carriers have developed diagnosis related guidelines (DRGs) designed to limit the scope and extent of treatment for specific conditions. All of these techniques reflect a fundamental tension at the heart of any economic system designed to increase access to health care; namely, that increasing access also increases costs, and that decreasing costs, except at the margins, has to involve some level or another of decreasing care.

By itself, the mere presence of insurance available for purchase doesn't solve the problem of access, however, though it does ameliorate it. There will always be a class of people who do not have insurance, either because they can't afford it, or they don't want to spend the money, or insurance companies refuse them coverage for a variety of reasons. For these individuals and families, the mere presence of insurance available for purchase does not necessarily translate into access, since they lack the means to pay for treatment out of pocket. Their access to care may in fact be worse in a system where insurance is generally available, since caregivers used to insurance reimbursement may have no incentive to accept uninsured, financially limited customers. In terms of providing care to all members of the community, this system may still fare relatively badly in terms of access, though better, probably, than the pure free market version examined earlier.

The introduction of insurance as part of the economic system changes health care in other ways. One of the ways it changes the system is by setting up an alternative financial power in the system, and that power can be used to determine or influence various aspects of the system. If insurance covers back surgery, but not chiropractic services, for example, we would expect to find many more back surgeons than chiropractors, so insurance coverage will affect what sorts of treatments are available, and also the number of practitioners offering them. One of the ways that HMOs were supposed to lower costs when they were first established was by setting standards of treatment that would be based on best practices research, eliminating ineffective treatments and thus bringing down the cost of health care as a whole.

But insurance companies could also limit access in other, less savory ways. Since they are concerned to keep costs down and their own profits high, they have a strong incentive to avoid paying claims if and when possible. Two methods of achieving this aim are, first, to avoid taking on people as customers who might require extensive medical treatment, and second, to avoid actually paying for the patients that they have taken on. Both of these methods are, of course, regularly encountered in the real world. Given that unregulated insurance companies are straightforward profit-oriented enterprises, and that the most direct way to increase profits is to deny claims, one would expect, and would find, that denial of claims and/or coverage is widespread and a serious problem with systems of this sort. One of the costs associated with an unregulated insurance system in any real-world system will be these sorts of unjust denials of care.

There is a very strong impetus for insurance companies to deny even legitimate claims when they believe that they can do so with impunity. Denial of claims in medical treatment is particularly tempting, because for many conditions, if treatment is denied for any length of time, the patient may die without treatment, and any further claims are also avoided. (Morbid, but true.) There is some evidence that insurance companies do engage in this type of behavior, though it is difficult to document how frequently it occurs. Concerns were raised at one point, for example, that some HMOs used retrospective denial of funding claims to deter 911 calls (Neely et al., 1999), while a more recent study of appeals of benefit denials at two HMOs found that a majority of appeals were successful, suggesting that many denials are inappropriate (Gresenz et al., 2011).

Rather remarkably, concerns of this sort about the problematic incentive structure of insurance companies themselves, and the serious cost to patients that can result, are often not addressed in any detail by proponents of a free market insurance system. To choose one egregious example, P.M. Booth and G.M. Dickinson, arguing that the UK should adopt a system more closely modeled on the US, spend several pages stipulating the ways that customers must be screened to prevent insurance companies from taking on too much risk, but never once mention a concern for regulation of the companies in order to protect the customers (Booth and Dickinson, 1998). Corporations are no more immune to immoral actions than are private individuals, and given the difference in power between a multi-million-dollar corporation and a middle-class individual, wrongdoing by the former should worry policymakers more than wrongdoing by the latter.

An ethics of care calls our attention to this power dynamic and its moral relevance. Power imbalances occur in any system of care provision, almost as a matter of logical necessity. When one party needs care and another is positioned to provide it, the latter stands in a position of power vis-à-vis the other. From the perspective of an ethics of care, that power differential in and of itself is not objectionable, but it does require moral scrutiny in terms of how the power is used. In the case of large insurance companies tasked with paying for care for sick and vulnerable individuals, there are at least two dangerous dynamics at work. The first I've already noted: there is a strong (and perverse) incentive to maximize profits by denying claims that, in the absence of strong regulation and oversight, results in widespread injustices and denials of care. But the incentive system is not the only problematic feature of this system. In addition to incentives, this system distances those making decisions about covering or denying claims from those who need care. This is one of the complaints made regularly by both patients and caregivers—that medical decisions are being made by 'some faceless bureaucrat' in an insurance office somewhere, totally removed from the reality of what denial means to the patient faced with no access to needed care, or to the caregiver, forced in to a situation where she knows that treatment exists and will work, but she cannot offer it to the patient because of insurance denials.

Both patient and caregiver feel the full brunt of this injustice; those perpetrating it are carefully removed to a distance that allows them to treat claims as nothing more than statistics and numbers. That distance is typical when power is being wielded against the interests of those it should serve. Because we are social beings, blatant denial of care generates enormous stress on most normal humans, and we frequently resort to distancing techniques to avoid the discomfort and to maintain our own sense of being decent moral agents. To the extent that this is built into the structure of insurance-based systems, it marks a very problematic aspect of that economic structure. It should not surprise us, then, to find that the combination of incentives and structural distance together generates a situation in which people do act in deeply unethical ways, leading to the major litigation many insurance companies now face from the attorneys general of several states.

These concerns are, in fact, part of the considerations that might move a society into the third possible economic system, that of a regulated insurance-based system. I'll discuss that shortly.

Based on the way that insurance systems function in the real world, further, we can make some reasonable assumptions about some of the drawbacks of any insurance system. I mentioned earlier the bureaucratization and complexity that seem inherent components of any unregulated insurance system. But the frustrations of caregivers go much deeper than just the stacks of paperwork and redundant information they are forced to submit. Worse, from their perspective, is the constant insertion of relatively arbitrary third parties into treatment decisions. A physician may be convinced because of the many cases that she has seen that the generic version of drug X simply doesn't work as well as the brand name version. There are a number of generics that are not subject to as strict quality control as the brand name product. When the dosages are not as accurate for the generic, it can make a difference for patients, particularly ones made more vulnerable by being on a number of other medications simultaneously, or being in weakened condition overall. But if an insurance company has decided that the generic is the one they will cover, then the physician's hand is forced—generic or nothing.

As I argued in Chapter 2, furthermore, the move to EBP has legitimated the notion of cost-effectiveness. But cost-effectiveness requires a very subjective assessment of what level of cost can legitimately be traded off against what level of effective treatment. When that decision is being made by (again) faceless bureaucrats in an insurance building somewhere, whose main concern (in good capitalist fashion) is protecting the stockholders' right to make a profit, the patient's well-being is unlikely to be served. In addition to cost-effectiveness guidelines, insurance companies often set treatment guidelines that are fairly rigid. For example, insurance will only cover intensive care for many patients for a set number of days or weeks, after which they must be transferred to a continuing care facility. In response, many physicians and nurses have learned to game the system, recording conditions that will generate justification for a longer stay, or tweaking diagnoses to meet insurance criteria.

From the caregiver's perspective, the need to twist diagnoses or manipulate the system in an attempt to get needed treatment for patients is extremely problematic. Since one of our criteria for analysis is the way that a given system shapes the caregiver's character, a system that demands caregivers choose either dishonesty or a failure to provide care is not a well-designed system. And when the limitations on care are arbitrary or even morally problematic, the strain on caregivers is even more troubling.

But while it is important to recognize that arbitrary restrictions on care are problematic, it is also important to note that any economic structure will have to put some restrictions on care. Resources are finite, and no realistic system can provide unlimited access to all the medical care anyone could use. The question that needs to be asked is whether the way that an unregulated insurance system limits care is more problematic, more detrimental to caregivers' character, or more likely to produce bad care altogether. And here the jury is out. Caregivers are often frustrated, it is true, and find themselves gaming the system, but comparing the level of these issues with that found in other systems requires a comparison with other options. All things considered, caregivers generally can provide better care in a system with insurance than in a straight fee-for-service system, in spite of the structural problems.

From the perspective of an ethics of care, a market-based insurance system is better than a complete free market system, but still has serious flaws in terms of access to care. While it can ensure broader access generally to medical care, it still leaves those unable to afford insurance without care.

Furthermore, the inherent tension that insurers face between maximizing profits or providing care is a structural problem that is extremely problematic. Add to this the fact that market-based insurance systems increase the distance between those who need care and those who have the authority to make decisions about who receives care, and the result is one that is ripe for ethical problems.

Overall, an unregulated insurance market has some drawbacks, but it does, all the same, offer some positives as well. It dramatically increases access to effective care over the purer free market system, and it can improve the level of care in cases where the insurer mandates that all caregivers in the system provide a particular standard of care (though this is counterbalanced to some extent by the incentive the system provides for insurers to define the standard of care in terms of least expensive rather than most effective). It is a system that protects some aspects of the caregiver/patient relationship by removing the most direct financial links between caregivers and patients. But the dynamics of the relationship leave patients vulnerable to exploitation by the insurance company, and provide little to no protection for consumers. For those and other reasons, in the contemporary world, many countries have adopted a system that maintains the basic structure of insurance but governs the relationship between insurers and customers with relatively strict government oversight.

State-Regulated Insurance Models

On the regulated insurance model, both customers and companies face government regulation, so this is a system that moves along the spectrum away from a free market toward a much higher level of state control. Citizens, on this model, are required to carry insurance, usually with some form of subsidy provided for lower income purchasers. Insurance providers are required to offer a particular range of coverage, and either the rates they can charge or the level of profit they can make is regulated (treating them, in effect, like utilities, rather than as independent businesses). Insurance companies are generally very limited in terms of denial of coverage; they are not allowed to exclude individuals with pre-existing conditions or to limit their customer base to the healthiest while excluding sicker patients from coverage. Lifetime caps on coverage are prohibited in many regulated insurance systems.

The majority of regulated insurance systems produce a two-tiered system of providing medical care because in most of them, wealthier citizens supplement the publicly provided insurance with private insurance. This issue has been particularly contentious in Canada, where extensive debates raged for several years about whether or not a province had to allow citizens to purchase private insurance. While the matter has been settled legally by the Supreme Court of Canada, which found that private citizens' rights would be unacceptably infringed if they were prevented from choosing to purchase such insurance, the ethical debate had not entirely subsided (Flood et al.,

2005). The Supreme Court's argument relied on the priority of individual liberty; the opposing side argued that allowing individuals to purchase private insurance would irretrievably weaken the public insurance system in ways that would be contrary to Canada's responsibility to provide for all citizens.

In terms of access, regulated insurance models in the real world have done a better job of ensuring access for the vast bulk of the population than the 'free market' system (Angell, 2008; American College of Physicians, 2008; Lasser et al., 2006), and also do a much better job at ensuring care for those with lower incomes (Schoen and Doty, 2004). (This is not surprising, as this is exactly what they are designed to do.) They generate this result while keeping expenditures much lower; Canadian life expectancy is two to three years longer than US life expectancy, while Canada spends about half as much per citizen on health care overall than does the US (Angell, 2008). In 2017, US per-capita health care expenses were estimated to be around $10,348, Canadian expenditures $4,752 (both in US dollars) (Sawyer and Cox, 2018).

From a purely economic perspective, the real-world track record of a free market insurance system, at least as practiced in the US, has little to recommend it in terms of value for money. The inefficiencies of the system may arise, in part, because of the quirks of the system (employer-provided health care, government programs that supplement the market systems, and legal requirements that people presenting at emergency rooms receive treatment regardless of ability to pay, for example), but most proponents of a market system of health care delivery do seem more driven by ideological commitment to libertarian economic principles than by empirical studies. Cost-to-outcome ratios, however, are only one part of the ethical examination of an economic system of health care delivery.

It is clear that a regulated insurance system will produce greater access to health care. This is not the only feature of health care that is ethically relevant, however. Measures of factors such as patient satisfaction would also seem relevant, as are the issues noted earlier concerning the ways that a system impacts the caregiver/patient relationship and the character of health care professionals themselves.

Accurate measurement of how people themselves rate the care they receive under any given system is difficult issue. The World Health Organization does publish comparative studies of various national health care systems, but uses expert evaluations rather than patient surveys to establish satisfaction, and as a recent study pointed out, the two do not always coincide. Whichever system is used, however, there is some evidence that patient satisfaction is relatively high in the US, even among the poor (Blendon et al., 2001), in ways that do not correlate with outcomes measurements (life expectancy, and so on). In one of the most widely cited studies, the Joint Canada/United States Survey of Health 2002–2003, US patients were more likely to be 'very satisfied' with their health care and their physician, while

Canadians were more likely to be 'somewhat satisfied,' even though on a number of specific measures (unmet health care needs, self-reporting as having poorer health), Americans were slightly worse off, on the whole, than Canadians (Sanmartin et al., 2004). (The numbers for insured Americans and Canadians are largely indistinguishable.) Living near the US/Canadian border, I am tempted to interpret some of these differences as cultural differences. (Many Canadians, even on their wedding day, are likely to rate themselves as doing somewhat okay rather than very okay, but my sample size is, I am sure, inadequate to the task.) All told, though, there does seem to be some suggestion that US citizens with insurance find their health care to be more satisfactory than do their neighbors to the north.

Turning to caregivers rather than patients, a similar ambiguity exists in trying to make international comparisons, especially for comparing physician job satisfaction. With respect to nurses, however, who represent the front line of patient care for a wide variety of treatments, the best conclusion to draw from the available evidence is that nurses around the world are experiencing stress and succumbing to burnout at rates that bode ill for patients in every health care system. A few statistics tell the story: in the US, 41% of nurses report high levels of dissatisfaction with their jobs; 43% score in the high burnout range. The numbers for Canada are marginally better (32.9%, 36%) but both are far higher than the average rate of dissatisfaction or burnout ranges for all other occupations (which tend to run in the 10% range) (Aiken et al., 2001). Germany was the only country reporting ranges lower than 20% on either measure. In this case, differences between systems of regulated and unregulated insurance seem to make little difference in job satisfaction; nurses in both cases are overworked, stressed out, and frustrated that they cannot offer adequate care to their patients.

Nurses, it seems to me, are the canary in the coal mine of medicine. In the acute care setting, they are at the front lines of patient care, interact with their patients for far more hours in the day, far more intensively, than any other caregiver, and the work they do has a tremendous effect on patient outcomes. Further, nursing as a profession has long been associated with altruistic care, generating expectations from both patients and nurses themselves that they will provide care that goes beyond mere physical attentiveness and responds to the emotional and social needs of the patients they care for (Reverby, 1987). Given this, one might expect that nurses would experience their job as rewarding and satisfying. Instead, nurses experience burnout and leave the profession in large numbers. One reason for this is the structure of job organization and reimbursement that has developed from the standard economic models, particularly the insurance-based models (both regulated and unregulated). Short-staffing, scheduling too few to nurses to provide adequate care for patients, for example, correlates strongly with nursing burnout (Boamah et al., 2017).

Because insurance reimbursement is regulated at a legislative level, it will funnel resources toward certain types of treatment and away from others. In particular, insurance covers diagnostic tests, specific procedures, surgeries, and the like—all easily specified concrete 'units.' This makes sense from an insurance company's perspective, because it makes reimbursement predictable and controllable. What it leaves out of coverage, or only offers low rates of coverage for, however, is the actual hands-on care that has traditionally been a central feature of nursing care. Health care workers (not just nurses, though they feel the brunt of it) regularly report that what they *don't* get paid for is spending time with a patient. Yet time spent, one on one, correlates very closely with good outcomes (Flocke, 2002; Papastavrou 2013). But time is an open-ended factor, and one that does not quantify nearly as neatly as diagnostic tests—there are no clear charts or percentile measurements at the end of spending some time with a patient. Further, time is very sensitive to individual differences: a good clinician spending time with a patient may produce quite different results than a bad one, and even the nature of caregiver/patient relationship can change the nature of the time spent.

What is true of time is even more true of some of the other aspects of good nursing care: time, attentiveness, and care itself are all amorphous (at least from the perspective of a budget officer) and hard to quantify. So, when budgets need to be cut, these are the factors that bear the brunt of the cuts, and the fact that they can't be easily quantified means that those who do value them (both caregivers and patients) often lack the means to argue for their effectiveness. It is almost impossible to demonstrate that this extra 15 minutes of talking resulted in that increase in patient well-being, though one can show that allowing room in schedules for these things increases patient well-being statistically.

There is a second dynamic at work in the tendency of insurance systems to squeeze out the essential components of good nursing care, and that is the fact that everyday care simply doesn't make exciting headlines. When an insurance carrier refuses treatments that are dramatic, potentially life-saving, and (of course) technologically interesting and expensive, the media finds the resulting human interest stories irresistible (see, for example, Kiser, 2010). But when an insurance company decides that it will only cover three days of skilled nursing care post-op for certain types of surgery, rather than the four to five days that most patients really need, it is hard to make a dramatic story out of the loss of a day. Most patients will probably survive; they'll just do so with a greater risk of infection, at greater cost to the family members who will have to try to substitute for skilled nursing care without training, and so on. Public opinion doesn't get mobilized when nursing care gets cut; it does when surgical intervention is cut.

The result of this dynamic is that insurance carriers, rather paradoxically, often are far more willing to cover extremely expensive, sometimes experimental treatments than they are to provide the basic care that far more people need. Cuts at the level of basic care go unnoticed; cuts to high-tech care get covered by major news services (Allen, 2011). And once the story has 'legs,' so to speak, it becomes the focus of legislation and money gets channeled to that particular cause, without much deliberation about how paying for that type of care will impact the rest of the system. But the money spent there has to come from somewhere, and as we've already seen, the 'somewhere' is frequently the more basic parts of health care, especially nursing care.

This produces an ever-increasing squeeze on nurses; their patients today are far sicker than they were 30 years ago, and they see more of them, for less time, than they used to. It thus becomes harder for them to do what they are actually educated to do: to care for a patient's needs holistically. The result is that nurses become overwhelmed, burned out, and exhausted (Flynn and Ironside, 2018; Chin et al., 2017). From the perspective of an ethics of care, I need hardly say, this whole dynamic is disastrous. It is also paradoxical, since insurance companies should be in the business of making decisions on the basis of cost-effectiveness. Basic care, including nursing care, is constantly cited as far more cost-effective than high-end, technologically driven procedures. But it is always worth remembering that even corporations devoted to calculating economic costs and benefits can find themselves acting in economically irrational ways due to the pressures of public opinion, internal systemic forces, and sheer inertia. For good or ill, economic analysis is not as determinative of policy as is often thought.

So just as there are both important positives to a free market system, along with serious negatives, both insurance-based systems likewise produce some extremely important results, particularly in their contributions to much wider access to medical care, while simultaneously producing side effects, intended or unintended, that are potentially damaging to care delivery and to caregivers themselves.

The Public Health Model

Furthest along our spectrum from a free market model is one that eliminates the third-payer/insurance company system and provides health care directly as a government service, much like public education. On this model, health care is considered a basic component of public services, and is provided for all citizens, much of it at no out-of-pocket cost or for a very low fee. Health care workers on this model are public servants, hired by and accountable to the government. As in the case of regulated insurance markets, individuals who want to can opt out of the system by purchasing private insurance that entitles them to a separate level of health care (much as parents in the US can choose to purchase private schooling for their children), though this remains controversial among ethicists because of the way it produces a two-tiered system of medical care.

All public health systems face some version of what Albert Weale calls 'an inconsistent triad' of commitments. Weale argues that the commitments implicit in a system of public health are: (1) that health care will be provided comprehensively (that is, it will offer a full range of treatments), (2) it will be provided freely (without undue barriers to anyone, whether financial or social), and (3) it will provide high quality care. The challenge is that it seems that "a system of health care can be comprehensive and freely available but not of high quality; or it can be high-quality and available to all, but not comprehensive; or it can be comprehensive and of high quality but not available to all" (Weale, 1998, p. 139). As a matter of fact, Weale does argue that it is possible for a public health system to meet all three of these to some degree, but his initial framing of the problem states the challenges of such a system admirably.

A public health system is designed to resolve the problem of access, and so the issues that arose for an unregulated insurance system or a free market system will not be characteristic of such a system. Care will be accessible to all. But there are costs to providing care for all, and any public system will have to figure out how to deal with them, one way or another. The first is not so much access overall, but timely access; the standard criticism of a public health system by free market proponents is the lack of immediate access, and the need to wait (for non-emergency services) for much longer periods of time than patients do in more market-oriented systems such as the US. This criticism is valid. Wait times in many publicly funded systems are significantly higher for a number of procedures, such as hip replacements and back surgeries. The wait times and deferrals of treatment reflect the fact that a system that provides coverage for all citizens will need to utilize resources strategically if it is not to bankrupt its citizens by high taxes, and one straightforward way to use resources carefully is to limit the number of (say) MR imagers, producing waits for the patients needing scans. The US, for example, performs more MRI scans and CT scans than most comparison countries in part because other systems limit the number of scanners available (Papanicolas et al., 2018), and while this probably indicates a level of over-utilization of resources, it does produce very short wait times for the procedure.

A second issue faced by public health systems is the question of which treatments will be offered, and what the limits to treatment will be. In political discourse, it is common to hear slogans such as "We need to meet all the health care needs of our citizens," but a public system will necessarily face constraints on what can be offered, due to the limits of the funding it has available. So, for example, up until the 1980s, the UK had an unofficial age limit of around 55 for referrals for dialysis (Schmidt, 1998), and since renal failure tends to be a disease of old age, this kept the number of people receiving dialysis very low (and, of course, concomitant costs lowered as well). While there are no officially stated national policies for age limits on procedures such as organ transplants, a recent survey found that of 71 renal centers surveyed in the UK, three had explicit age cutoffs for kidney transplants (at 75 years) and about a third of the centers did not have formal assessment criteria, leaving open the possibility that elderly patients were less likely to be referred for transplants (Pruthi et al., 2018).

Given the ever-increasing cost of health care and the constant spiral of newer and more expensive technologies in health care, any public health system will face the difficulty that it is asked (by a public informed by the media of every new and exciting technique in medicine) to continue to provide all that can be done for a problem with an ever-more-limited supply of tax dollars. And if those tax dollars are not to disappear into (in Daniel Shapiro's expressive phrase) "the equivalent of a black hole that sucks out resources devoted to all other goods" (Shapiro, 1998, p. 105), then some form of rationing, or of limiting expenditures (if that phrasing sounds less contentious) must be found.

Public health systems often have a committee that reviews various treatment protocols and approves only those that have a certain cost-effectiveness. In the UK, the review board is the National Institute for Health and Clinical Excellence (NICE), and they are tasked with setting the rules for what treatments will be covered and which won't be. Critics of these systems, like Shapiro, argue that two features of committees such as NICE make them problematic on egalitarian grounds. First, these committees deliberate in private, and though their policies may be made public, there is rarely much transparency in the process by which they reach those policies. Second, nationally constructed policies tend to produce results that favor the upper and middle classes, both because their membership is usually drawn from those echelons, and also because, whatever the limits they set are, the wealthier and better-educated citizens will be better able to work the system to get the treatments they need (Shapiro, 1998). Because of the lack of transparency, and the capacity that the better-off have to game the system, it has been argued, a market system that allows consumers to make their own choices about what should (or need not) be included in insurance coverage allows for a far more individualized, less monolithic set of choices, and this is more egalitarian than a system that sets one policy by which all are required to work.

The question of whether a market-regulated system is or is not more egalitarian than a policy-regulated system depends crucially on whether one's egalitarianism is an egalitarianism of resources or of outcomes, and that is a question I cannot resolve here. Shapiro's question is whether the provision of a one-size-fits-all health system (with, presumably, a second tier accessible to those with money and education) necessarily entails that the health care accessible to the poorest will be of a lower quality than that to which others have access (the answer, if one is honest, is yes, almost by definition). But perhaps the question he needs to be asking is a different one: whether the care accessible to the poor on such a system, inferior though it may be to the care available to those wealthier and more educated, is worse altogether than the care those same poor would have access to on a free market system;

and that question is a good deal harder to answer, though there are good reasons to think the answer is no.

Publicly funded health systems do face one particularly serious threat to the caregiver/patient relationship that Shapiro identifies, and that is the tendency of caregivers to ration unconsciously rather than have to inform patients that a particular type of care is unavailable for economic reasons. Caregivers generally do not want to explicitly inform patients that there are treatments available that could cure an illness or prevent death, but for economic reasons they are unavailable. Shapiro argues that under conditions of limited economic availability, what caregivers are likely to do is simply not mention that the unavailable treatments even exist, or, if they are mentioned, refer to them as 'contra-indicated' or as unlikely to be of benefit (Shapiro, 1998). And this seems likely, if not in every case, in a sufficiently broad range of cases to be of concern.

Under such conditions, rationing will take place, but it will fly under the radar in such a way that the patients whose care is rationed may not know that they are experiencing treatment denial. And as Shapiro reminds us, this rationing will be likely to fall most heavily on the poor and uneducated; the educated will be far more likely to seek out a second opinion, ask about alternative ways of phrasing a diagnosis so as to gain access to a wider range of treatments, and so on. Rationing under a national health care system also takes place due to limits to the amount of money available at any given time within the system itself; NICE, for example, may hold that up to three rounds of in vitro fertilization (IVF) are available for couples dealing with infertility, but somewhat arbitrary screening criteria and lengthy waits for treatment create limits to who gains access to IVF (Ledger and Skull, 2009; Lord et al 2009).

Conclusion

In the course of this chapter, I have not examined every possible twist on the economic structures underlying contemporary medicine. I have not, for example, discussed medical savings accounts, a favorite topic for economists of a libertarian stripe. It seems to me that these savings accounts are generally a modification of some form of insurance policy—either they function to allow an individual to purchase insurance, or they function as insurance against at least some expenditures in medicine, albeit perhaps a rather minimalistic sort of insurance. But they face the same questions as insurance-based systems (society needs to decide whether to make such accounts mandatory, or not, and if not, whether to allow/require the indigent to die for lack of funds, and so on). And they do not obviate the need to decide whether or not to regulate insurance—that is an issue that can go either way, regardless of savings plans. Most likely, there are other possibilities that various theorists have put forward that I have neglected as well, not because I dislike them, but because this chapter is quite long enough as it is.

However, in looking at even the range of possibilities offered in this chapter, we can draw some conclusions about how economics affects care, and the first thing we need to recognize is that there is no perfect system. Regardless of the economic structure a society adopts, there will be trade-offs, and because we are talking about health care, those trade-offs will take a toll on people in terms of pain and suffering, in terms of their inability to get care that would be of real benefit to them, and in terms of whether or not they continue to live. The most frustrating part of thinking about health care economics is the way it brings home our finitude. We cannot provide everything to everyone without bankrupting the system, and if the system goes bankrupt, then care will truly become a scarce commodity. Our only options are to choose among the various systems (or variants thereof) and try to mitigate the drawbacks of each as best we can.

I have, in this chapter, pointed out some of the reasons why there is no utopian solution to the economics of health care. The available treatments are simply too expensive and work too well to be able to make them available to absolutely everyone; at some point, we will have to decide which treatments to support and which to consider a luxury that the wealthy can purchase for themselves, but which we cannot ensure for everyone. And, further, to the extent that we decide to spread access more broadly across the population, we will increasingly find ourselves faced with fewer resources spread more thinly among a larger population.

Given those constraints, the perils of trying to think through the economics of health care in the midst of contentious politically polarized contexts are enormous. Any attempt to reign in the spiraling costs of health care leave people open to charges of trying to 'kill grandma' or set up 'death panels'; attempts to extend care to a wider range in the population are criticized for being fiscally irresponsible and profligate. The general tendency of the media is to look for the inflammatory stories about patients who lack access to organ transplants or expensive technology, but almost never to spend time reporting on the need for basic care or the difficulty of making decisions about what not to fund.

Some sociologists argue that when we humans think about complicated matters (such as the provision of health care), we begin with a set number of story templates, each of which is structured with a set of values that largely determine how we reason in any given situation. So, one of the standard story templates is the notion that any individual facing death or serious illness should be saved, if there is some treatment that could save him or her. Further, they should be saved regardless of cost. (This storyline does not just occur in medicine. We see similar reasoning when, say, hikers get lost on a mountain in a blizzard—helicopters should be sent out, regardless of expense, and regardless of risk to the rescuers.)

The 'heroic rescue' story, however, only gets activated when there is a single, identifiable individual who becomes a cause célèbre. When the issue concerns a class of individuals (children needing vaccinations, for example), then the storylines blur. For some this triggers the 'irresponsible parents neglecting their kids' storyline, while for others it activates the 'we need to take care of our own' storyline. When the issue is even more amorphous (nursing burnout), there is no clear storyline because it is too hard to pinpoint responsible parties, and too difficult to put a face to the problem, and so people shrug and simply pay no attention, nurses leave in droves, and patients get shorter and shorter shrift in hospitals.

An ethics of care offers one way of calling our attention to the 'care' component of medicine, rather than focusing solely on the 'treatment' component. Health care is fundamentally a system of offering care to one particularly vulnerable group in society, and that needs to be the central focus of our debates about how to fund health care, how much to provide, and what particular aspects of health care we should emphasize. The current tendency to frame health care as a commodity, unfortunately, makes a care focused analysis difficult.

From the perspective of care theory, health care and other practices of providing care to meet people's basic needs cannot be treated as one commodity among others. As Daniel Engster argues in *The Heart of Justice*, the provision of care is a core aspect of human life. Without care, human life cannot exist or flourish. For this reason, the provision of care cannot be treated as merely one component of the social fabric, to be traded off against other values such as the production of wealth. Instead, care must be, as his title indicates, at the heart of any just social system (2007, p. 59). While health care, like any large-scale social practice, needs to be structured in ways that are economically sustainable, it cannot be adequately analyzed if it is treated as merely one commodity among others, and this rules out any systems of providing care that are completely market driven.

The complexity of trying to provide care in the context of market driven-economic systems is generated by a number of factors. One of the most basic is the tendency for care work in particular to be limited as a way of minimizing costs. As Engster notes, "Competition among health care providers creates incentives to minimize hospital stays, limit the clinical options of doctors, and substitute unlicensed 'care technicians' for registered nurses" (2007, p. 131). There are strong incentives for health care systems to offload the actual work of care to semi-skilled or unskilled providers, especially to family members who are expected—sometimes even forced—to provide that work at a fairly heavy cost to their own time and career options (Folbre, 2013; Glen, 2010). I have mentioned numerous other factors earlier in this chapter, including the problem of unpredictability of need and enormous expenses for many treatments, and the like.

While I do not advocate returning to a pure free market system in health care, I do think there are valuable lessons to be learned from imagining that scenario. The first is that a market system allows people to seek out a broad range of caregivers. Contemporary medicine tends to operate with a model of physician-focused medical treatment as the central task of all medical care, and a libertarian analysis reminds us that many aspects of care could be provided by a range of caregivers. Free market analyses also offer valuable reminders that the resources for providing care are not unlimited. Both of these are important considerations for any analysis of the economic structures of health care.

But because it is clear that from the perspective of care theory, the economic structures of health care need to be organized so that basic care is available to those who need it, a pure free market system is not ethically justifiable. It does seem reasonable to assume, however, that there is a range of systems which could be adopted, so long as they meet the basic criteria for a decent level of health care. Two criteria in particular set the standard for an adequate system: the provision of a reasonable level of health care for all, and a system that ensures that those who provide that care—particularly those who are in the trenches, so to speak, providing the hands-on, day-to-day care that is vital to health care—must themselves be provided with adequate wages and working conditions in order to avoid exploitation and burnout (Tronto, 2013; Kittay, 1999). The second of these—decent pay and working conditions for all who provide care—is not an insurmountable issue. But the first represents a more difficult set of choices and deliberations.

As medical technology continues to develop, the cost of providing life-saving and health preserving treatments to everyone who needs them will outstrip the resources available to pay for it. Many of those who study health care economics argue that we have already moved to the point of promising a level of care to all that cannot be sustained (Fleck, 2009). We must, at some point, begin to articulate the limits of what can reasonably be expected in terms of health care, either in terms of what the public coffers should provide, or in terms of what can be provided through some form of market mechanism, with (presumably) adequate regulation to resolve problems of exploitive insurance companies and the like. None of the systems discussed here dictate the level of health care that a decent society must provide, but all face this same dilemma.

An ethics of care points our attention, first and foremost, to two things: to actual care (rather than to the provision of as much technological magic as can be afforded), and to the relationship between provider and patient. The quandaries of economics have generated a number of problematic tensions for the latter. Whether it is physicians lying to get care not covered by insurance, or nurses suffering burnout as their ranks are stretched thinner and thinner by funding cuts, or physicians failing to even mention the existence of a treatment that could change the course of a patient's illness because it is unlikely to be funded—in each of these cases, the economic structure corrupts the relationship in important ways. One basic principle an ethics of care would support is that of favoring economic systems that allow for the most transparent funding systems possible to avoid this corrosion of the caregiver/client relationship.

Having noted this, however, we must still conclude that economic limitations are real, and we cannot make them go away by wishing for a world without limits (Groenhout, 2015). Whatever system we choose to set up in our various societies will either leave some individuals without access to care (because they lack insurance, for example) or limit the amount of care provided to some individuals (because the system lacks the resources to offer them). This is not a pleasant conclusion to reach. Physicians do not want to be told that they cannot offer adequate care to patients; health care systems do not want to be told that their eagerness to provide high-tech treatment has deleterious effects on patients because it results in a nursing shortage. In both cases, the motives of those responsible are good motives (hence the anger and personal insult they often take when these forces are pointed out). But the unwillingness to be honest about these dynamics ensures that they will continue, and makes it likely that they will be exacerbated. So, one economic principle that an ethics of care endorses (like many other ethical theories) is that of transparency and openness about how decisions are made, who has the responsibility for making them, and the like. While this cannot by itself resolve issues of economic limitations, it at least avoids the problem of having unaccountable, anonymous decision-makers.

A second emphasis that is natural for an ethics of care is a preference for relationships over technology. No ethical theory can resolve the problem of finite resources. But, as will be discussed in the next chapter, technology has a way of driving health care decisions than needs to be resisted. This is not because technology is evil—it is desirable precisely because it is so effective. But technology captures our attention and often becomes the focus of medical decisions, when what patients frequently need is care offered by individuals who are willing to focus on them. Technology can become a substitute for attention in problematic ways, and an ethics of care reminds us that personal relationships are of central importance during the hard transitions in life. To the extent that our economic resources are directed toward supporting and protecting personal relationships rather than solely providing access to various expensive treatments, we may find that more careful use of resources need not undermine care.

Notes

1 A system is efficient in the economic sense if it achieves the highest possible level of production and services for the lowest cost. Economic efficiency is solely a measure of how efficiently the monetary inputs are utilized, not a measure of whether (for example) natural resources are used wisely or time is used in an efficient manner.

2 The issue of how consumers are to gain access to adequate information is one of the more vexing questions for proponents of free market economics. If government programs are needed to investigate and disseminate information, then a true free market requires a relatively strong set of government systems, an outcome generally disliked by the most fervent proponents of the free market. Without such government programs, however, consumers are at such a disadvantage in making

decisions that their decisions about what to purchase simply cannot achieve efficiency in any reasonable way. Imagine, for example, an average middle-class consumer with high blood pressure trying to decide whether the low-salt diet her doctor recommends would be better than the expensive medicine offered by the pharmaceutical companies with glossy advertising and claims of miraculous cures. And, unlike decisions about purchasing cars, clothes, or houses, poor decisions about medical matters can actually kill a person, so the stakes are high, the information inaccessible and perhaps unintelligible to the average consumer, and disinformation widespread and extremely persuasive.

3 My point here is not that the costs are inappropriate. Basic economic analysis suggests that the benefits of medical treatment outweigh the costs, using standard quality-adjusted life year (QALY) criteria for calculating benefits (Cutler and McClellan, 2001). But while the personal benefits of many interventions outweigh the (economic) costs in the abstract; that does not in and of itself determine whether society as a whole can afford to provide those benefits.

4 Care and the Technological Imperative

In earlier chapters, the issue of technology and its place in contemporary medicine came up at several junctures. The change from conceptualizing knowledge in terms of clinical judgment to an evidence-based paradigm is reliant in numerous ways on the prevalence of computerized search engines and ready access to research on the internet. Patient access to information also drives technological change as knowledge generates demand. In terms of economic forces in health care, the soaring increase in technological prowess that characterizes contemporary medicine is one of the driving forces for the rapid increase in the cost of medicine, and so a contributing factor to the intractable trade-offs discussed in the previous chapter on economic structures.

Given how central technological change is to these other issues in health care, it seems worthwhile to spend some time thinking about technology itself and how it functions. Technology has changed medicine in fundamental ways over the past 50 years (and even more fundamentally if we look at the last 100 years). The differences range from enormous increases in basic capacities such as the switch from x-rays to MRIs, to new surgical techniques, to developing technologies of genetic medicine. As capacities change, changes occur to the experiences and expectations of patients, as well.

The way that medicine has changed can be seen if we compare a few basic aspects of medical care, thinking about what the limits of medicine were in the 1970s compared to the current situation. In the 1970s, for example, x-rays were the best visualizing tool available. The first MRI image of a living subject (a clam) was taken in 1973, and the first human MRI in 1977 (and it took five hours). Today, MRIs are standard equipment, almost completely supplanting x-ray technology in many areas because of a higher degree of resolution and the capacity for three-dimensional images (Roberts, 2006). And the presence of MRIs generates yet more technological breakthroughs such as the development of micro-surgery techniques using MRI guidance.

MRIs are wonderful technology; they are also costly technology. A new MRI costs between $1.5 and $3 million (plus the construction of an MRI suite that can easily cost another half million dollars). For comparison, x-ray scanners can be had for as little as $5,000.

In the 1960s and 1970s, kidney failure became treatable for the first time with the development of dialysis (Blagg, 2007). Today, kidney transplants are the preferred treatment for renal failure. The first successful human kidney transplants were performed between identical twins in the 1950s, but until surgical techniques improved and anti-rejection medications were developed, the procedure could not be used as a general treatment for renal failure. In 1980 in the US, there were about 7,500 kidney transplants; by 2007, the number was over 17,000 (NKUDIC 2011), and it continues to climb, limited only by shortages in donated kidneys. Unlike many other new technologies in medicine, kidney transplants are cheaper than dialysis as well, initially costing far more, but with a break-even time of about two and a half years, after which the transplant costs (primarily anti-rejection medications) cost less than a quarter of the cost of dialysis (University of Maryland, 1999).

Medical responses to infertility, likewise, have changed radically in this time period. The first child conceived via in vitro fertilization (IVF) was born in 1978, generating huge media outcry, threats of *Brave New World* genetic engineering, and stern warning from clerics about the dangers of 'playing God.' Today, according to the US Centers for Disease Control and Prevention (CDC, 2016), it is estimated that approximately 1% of all infants born in the US are the result of some form of assisted reproductive techniques, more than 61,000 babies in a given year. The average round of IVF is usually estimated to run somewhere between $10,000 and $15,000, and ratios of births to cycles of IVF (which vary due to a number of factors, including the age of the potential mother, other health-related conditions, and cause of infertility) can vary from 30% to 60% success rates (all statistics from advancedfertility.com). Techniques available and in regular use in infertility clinics include a whole range of procedures. The most basic is the now-standard IVF, in which egg and sperm are obtained from parents, placed together in a petri dish to allow fertilization to occur (it is hoped) with the resulting embryo (or embryos) then inserted into the woman's uterus. (Some multiple births are a result of inserting large numbers of embryos all at once, a technique some clinics use to increase their ratios of cycles to live births.) But allowing egg and sperm to take their own time in fertilization has become passé; many clinics now use intracytoplasmic sperm injection (ICSI) as a standard adjunct to IVF, since when the problem is low sperm motility, the injection of sperm into egg raises the number of embryos produced. (ICSI has not been extensively tested in animals, so we do not know whether the injection of low-motility sperm may result in a higher than normal ratio of abnormalities in the embryos so produced.) IVF also allows for a range of alternative reproductive decisions, whether the use of a surrogate, or the use of purchased sperm or eggs or embryos.

These three very different types of technology (MRIs, organ transplantation, IVF) represent the sorts of changes that medical practice has undergone in the past 50 or so years, driven by technological changes that are truly marvelous. Medicine today has the capacity to do things, routinely, that in years past were only dreamed of, and because we can do them, we do. One of the main reasons why the cost of health care has risen so tremendously is precisely because medical technology allows health care professionals to do so much more than they could do in the past. And because so much more can be done, the assumption is that it all must be done, and one consequence is the soaring cost of health care. But economic reasons are not the sole reason for concerns about new technologies. The concern, from a care perspective, focuses more on the issue of how technological innovations change relationships, especially (in this book) the relationships between caregiver and patient. As Howard Brody notes:

> We humans . . . are by nature tool-makers and tool-users. Our tools can have a major impact on the world we inhabit. Included within that impact is the reflexive impact that the use of the tool can have on ourselves and how we view ourselves. Once we have deployed certain types of tools, we are no longer capable of seeing ourselves as *not* using such tools.
>
> (Brody, 2009, p. 204)

The technologies we develop do not just impact economic structures, nor are their effects limited to the health benefits and costs they generate. They also change our understanding of what it means to live a 'normal' human life, and of the ways that relationships are constructed. These social consequences are vitally important for health care.

Having noted this, we can also note that there have been some technological developments that have not generated much uptake. Male (pharmaceutical) contraceptives, for example, have not been widely adopted. The disjunct between standard discourses of masculinity and hormonal regulation of fertility generates an enormous barrier to the adoption of this sort of technology (Oudshorn, 2004; Terry and Braun, 2011). Cochlear implants, likewise, are highly controversial because they are seen by many in the deaf community as an attack on deaf culture, and as indicative of "the desire of a majority culture to impose its language and values on the deaf rather than modify its institutions to take account of the perspective and needs of members of another culture" (Sparrow, 2005, p. 135). But these cases are striking in part because they are rather exceptional when it comes to medical technology. In both cases, the technology threatens a deep sense of identity, and because of this it has generated resistance, but when that threat is missing, it is rare that new technologies are rejected.

The majority of new technological capacities in medicine tend instead to generate the opposite reaction—that when we can do things, we feel we must do them—and it takes on particular force in the context of medicine because the stakes are so high for people's lives. Medicine deals with life-and-death matters, with reproduction and basic functionality and fighting off life-threatening illnesses. In that context, it is not surprising that technology is a tremendously powerful force, and one that needs careful analysis in terms of how it structures the delivery of health care today. To do that, I want to begin with what is called the technological imperative: once technology is in place, there is a tendency for people to think that because technology makes it possible for us to do something, we therefore must do it.

The Technological Imperative

It is worth spending a few pages thinking about how the technological imperative functions, and to what extent it drives our thinking and our practice as either patients or as practitioners in the health care field. In all three of the cases mentioned earlier—MRIs, dialysis and kidney transplants, and IVF—the presence of the technology makes its use appear mandatory. MRI scans are thus used even when x-ray technology is as effective and far less expensive (Moore et al., 2009). To pick another example, the largest growing group of patients receiving dialysis is the very elderly (aged 75 and older), in spite of the fact that outcomes for this age cohort include high rates of multiple complications, frequent and lengthy hospital stays, and five-year survival rates in one study as low as 2.4% (Munshi et al., 2001). In the case of IVF, infertile couples frequently find themselves on what one researcher has termed the 'infertility treadmill' (Harwood, 2007) because of the difficulty of deciding to stop treatment once it has been started. But this dynamic extends to other parts of health care, as well.

The assumption that because certain procedures are possible, they must be adopted, is a driving force in some of the most ethically complicated arenas of medicine, particularly in the context of research on new medical procedures and pharmaceuticals. All medical research is ethically complex because it sets up a potential conflict between the good of the individual patient and the more general good of increasing knowledge and benefitting the population at large. Medical practice is supposed to be conducted for the good of the individual patient. Research is conducted in order to get generalizable data to help future patients. Early stage medical research, then, is not conducted primarily for the good of an individual patient. Stage one trials in particular are performed in order to get information for medical practice in general, not for the benefit of the individuals who undergo the tests.

In recognition of this fact, anyone conducting research on human subjects must first subject their research proposal to an oversight board (usually an internal review board [IRB] or an ethics committee) which will review the proposal to ensure that first, it poses no unacceptable risk to participants, and second, that the structure of the proposed study is such that anyone being used as an experimental subject will be fully informed of the risks and potential consequences of the study. In order for a research protocol to pass an IRB review, the researcher is required to fully inform any participants of the nature of the study, the possible risks, and the like, and also to make it clear to research subjects that they can exit the study at any time. Researchers may assign a portion of the subjects randomly to a treatment protocol that might be completely ineffective or might have negative side effects. Early stage clinical trials are designed to test what levels of therapies are safe for use, and are not designed to benefit participants. Informed consent is a necessary safeguard because it is vital for both researchers and subjects to recognize clearly that an experiment is not the same thing as treatment.

Yet recent studies of people who sign up to be experimental subjects for various cancer treatments suggest that in spite of all these safeguards, patients still expect that participating in an experimental treatment program will be for their own benefit (Joffe et al., 2001; Coyne et al., 2003; Cox et al., 2006). This mistaken expectation is so common it has been given a name—the therapeutic misconception—and has been the focus of a number of clinical studies and ethical analyses (Goldberg, 2011; Koh et al., 2012). What is interesting about the dynamic set up in these cases is that the patient's own response to participation in the trial (I am signing up for an experimental protocol because I have to try everything that might help) is directly at odds with the information she or he has been given in the consent form. While the patients in these cases are informed at one level, at another level, a deeper emotional one, they are not acting on the information they have been given, but on quite a different set of beliefs.

Health care functions in a context structured by a deep faith in technology. Medical technology is seen as a powerful force, offering protection and cure for illness and death—two of humanity's deepest fears. And because so much medical technology has done amazing things, and because the medical field is one that is structured to benefit patients, faith in technology seems warranted in this context in a way it is not in others. Technological changes in other fields (manufacturing, computers, food production) frequently generate obvious side effects and conflicts of interest (pollution, privacy concerns, nutritionally questionable practices). In just the three medical cases mentioned earlier, however, technological interventions have improved so drastically that it is hard not to assume that the newer and more complex is always better. But this faith in technological fixes often blinds us to the costs and negatives of technological interventions.

MRIs do offer far better clarity and imaging than x-rays can, but the more widely they are used, the more expensive health care becomes. In the prior chapter, we noted the way that the choice to use expensive technology can come with a hidden cost—money spent to pay for the multiple MRI machines we currently use is money that must come from somewhere, in an increasingly expensive and constrained health care environment. And the cuts that are made to pay for newer and more expensive machines are often made to the less technological but no less important parts of health care: nursing staff, physician's time, hands-on care. Obviously, newer technologies need not always lead to higher expenses. Kidney transplants offer a clear case of a technological and surgical development that lowers costs (compared to dialysis) overall. Determining which technological changes generate sufficient benefit to patients to be worth implementing, which save money in the long run, and which do neither requires that we distance ourselves from the worship of technology that is so easy to slip into in the health care context.

The way we frame technology is particularly striking in end of life care. The increasing use of dialysis in the very elderly is a classic example of this: it is a practice that increases costs; increases the time an elderly individual must spend in the hospital, often in the disorienting context of an ICU; and does so with only marginal benefits in terms of additional years of life. But because the capacity is available, it must be used, regardless of how it impacts an individual's life or how it contributes to the economic pressures of the contemporary health care context.

As Daniel Callahan has argued, the close connection between how technology is understood and the mistaken notion that we can 'conquer death' or somehow eliminate mortality results in practices of end of life care that are often inhumane, wildly expensive, and largely useless in terms of any attainable goals (Callahan, 2009). We place too much hope in technology in the first place; in the context of thinking about death, our faith becomes essentially religious in nature. I will return to this topic in the final chapter of this book, on the ends of medicine and particularly on how our framing of what the point of medicine is affects practices like end of life care. For now, however, my focus is on how technology functions in our thinking, and my strong sense is that there is an unspoken, very powerful, quasi-religious faith that drives much of our reasoning, a faith that the miraculous power of some new technology will preserve us, and protect us from death itself.

The reason I am spending time detailing the way that the technological imperative functions, below the level of much of conscious thought, generating the assumption that technology is salvific, is that addressing a mythic structure of this sort cannot simply address the logical inconsistencies and false beliefs it generates, it must generate awareness of how the myth functions and identify its results in policies and practices of care. And on this issue Callahan's work has been invaluable, particularly his discussions of how end of life care is driven by technological developments in ways that can be tremendously detrimental to patients—the very people medical care exists to help.

Callahan notes that the technological imperative is behind much of the rhetoric that expresses what is going on in medicine and medical research. He cites William Haseltine's comment that "death is a series of preventable diseases" as one example of the way that contemporary research incorporates a version of the technological imperative that grounds the conviction that technology and research can do away with death altogether (Callahan,

1992). But, as Callahan goes on to point out, while it does make sense for a research agenda to focus on early and preventable deaths, it does not make sense to assume that what medical research should focus on is the elimination of death altogether. There are two fundamental reasons why it doesn't make sense. The first is that mortality is, as a matter of fact, part of our biological condition. The second is that the rhetoric of death as the enemy to conquer produces the sorts of 'care' that no one should have to undergo at the end of life: fragile 90-year-olds being resuscitated over and over, enduring shocks and broken ribs, because hospital policies require that cardiopulmonary resuscitation (CPR) be given unless there is an explicit do not resuscitate (DNR) order in the patient's file; weak and confused late-stage Alzheimer's patients spending weeks in the ICU because they can't be stabilized enough to return to a skilled care facility; the travesty of the political circus that arose over the Schiavo case[1]. (These are my examples, not Callahan's.) In all of these cases, we find individuals whose dying processes become prolonged agony, either for the individual or for the family. So long as conquering death is the main focus of medical technology, the patient actually undergoing the treatments and protocols is not really the focus of the medical care; if they were, our efforts would be geared toward providing them the best possible care in the last stages of their life.

One final aspect of the myth of saving technology should also be noted. Technological solutions to health problems are often (though not always) difficult, expensive, and fit well into a narrative of perseverance against all odds. It is generally the case, as noted in Chapter 2, that people find it easier to remember individual stories than statistical concepts (Betsch et al., 2011; Winterbottom et al., 2008; Williams, 2006). Technological marvels like organ transplants offer us individual faces of people miraculously saved from death by some technological miracle. Less exciting and low-tech procedures, such as vaccines, clean water, and basic instruction about ante-natal care for inexperienced mothers do not generate such stories of individual salvation—anyone saved through these methods is a statistical individual, not a particular person. We can document that various people do better—we can document that numerous people do better—when they have access to clean water, but we cannot identify the specific people who didn't catch dysentery, and didn't die. We just know that rates are lower.

This disparity between memorable individual cases and forgettable general statistics makes it politically difficult to limit the use of technology in health care; it also makes it harder to adequately fund the boring preventative care that is often the most economically effective. As an example, consider the national furor that arose in the US when Arizona, attempting to limit Medicaid expenditures, chose to deny funding for transplants for all patients older than 21. Within the space of only about four months, the policy was reversed due to the outrage and media attention the policy generated. Newspapers and television shows were full of stories about two individuals, in particular, who died after failing to have funding for transplant operations approved through Medicaid (Allen, 2011). During the same time period, Nebraska eliminated Medicaid funding for prenatal care for undocumented aliens. News reports at the time claimed that at least five babies died as a result of the cuts (Young, 2011). No national news agencies reported on the issue. Cuts to prenatal care do not have the same dramatic impact as the refusal of dramatic technological resources, even though they can have a greater impact overall on both life and health.

In summary, then, the technological imperative, in structuring the way we think about medicine, focuses our attention on staving off death at all costs, while failing to pay attention to the very real needs of the patient that go far beyond that single focus. It also prevents us from thinking realistically about the limits of medical resources: the language of salvation from death is so powerful that any attempt to limit what we spend on particular treatments and new technologies is always justified—after all, we need to save lives, and technology (remember the underlying assumptions) does just that. The fact that paying for that technology shunts resources from treatments that may be more effective in saving lives is obscured by the idolatry of technology. And, finally, it feeds into a particular narrative in medicine—the narrative of the heroic individual doing battle against the forces of evil—in ways that can make it hard to think clearly about how health care should be structured.

Ethical Problems Generated by the Technological Imperative

From the perspective of an ethics of care, the way that technology functions in our thinking generates a number of problematic ethical consequences. The issues with which I began this chapter—MRIs, dialysis and kidney transplants, and IVF—offer a helpful set of situations for thinking about what these problems are and why they arise. And, as a reminder, I chose these cases precisely because they are not particularly extreme or unusual, but are, instead, fairly standard medical uses of technology. There are three sets of ethical problems that are particularly central in this context: resource allocation, dehumanization of medical care, and unintended consequences. I'll deal with each of these in turn.

Before I do so, however, a reminder. While this section will discuss ethical issues that are raised by new technologies, the argument is not that technological change is bad and we should attempt to slow or reverse the trend toward the development of the technologies. Technological change can be wonderful and enormously beneficial. But it is precisely because it has such powerful potential that it is easy to slip into assuming that it always generates positive change, and always must be implemented. What I want to challenge is the unthinking adoption of technological change, not technology *simpliciter*.

Resource Allocation

Resources are finite in health care, and when money, time, and hospital space are devoted to any one set of programs, those resources are not available for other uses. Consider the case of organ donation, and the way that developments in the technological prowess with which we can transplant organs has created an automatic assumption that transplantation should be a standard part of medical treatment in the contemporary world.

Organ transplants are expensive, but there are tremendous variations across the spectrum of transplants. Kidneys are among the least expensive transplants and among the most cost-effective. A kidney transplant is less expensive than ten years of dialysis (averages range from around $20,000–50,000 for the surgery, with around $2,000–3,000 for anti-rejection drugs for each year thereafter), and the ten-year survival rate is currently over 85% (including the statistics for both live donation and cadaver donation). Studies have consistently found that transplants of kidneys is better for the patient's quality of life and is less expensive that home dialysis, and less expensive yet than in-hospital dialysis (Howard et al., 2009; Asgeirsdóttir et al., 2009; Winkelmayer et al., 2002). Liver transplants are generally considered the most expensive transplants, with first-year costs (including surgery and follow-up care) running around $577,000 (Bentley and Phillips, 2017). With livers, there is nothing comparable to dialysis as an alternative treatment; transplants are generally the only therapy available, so it is difficult to evaluate cost-effectiveness other than in QALYs (quality adjusted life years) or DALYs (disability-adjusted life years), both measures often derided by critics for 'putting a dollar value on life' and for systematically discounting certain types of lives (of the elderly and people with disabilities, for example) (Anand and Hanson, 2004). For some specific types of conditions, alternatives are available; for early stage hepatocellular carcinoma, for example, surgeons have used either early treatment (either chemotherapy or radiofrequency ablation) or have waited for the cancer to reach sufficient size for the patient to be put on a transplant recipient list (Naugler and Sonnenberg, 2010). (Livers are in such short supply that conditions have to be quite dire before one is placed on the recipient list; this has the paradoxical effect of increasing costs and lowering survival rates, since sicker patients respond less well to the rigors of transplantation and subsequent anti-rejection drugs.) Early treatment was considerably more cost-effective in this particular case than transplantation. Though the survival rates of both procedures differed only in terms of months (averaging a bit over five years in both cases), early treatment is far less expensive than transplantation.

With the advent of bioengineering, researchers are now investigating the possibility of creating livers from the patient's own cells, which would allow for an autologous transplant (that is, a transplant of the patient's own tissue). On the one hand, this would be wonderful news for the many patients who will never receive a donor liver. On the other hand, the projected costs for bioengineering a liver are $9.7 million (Habka et al., 2015). Liver transplant technology offers as clear an example of any of the need to actually consider what are the reasonable limits to extending life, because this level of expenditure on a single individual, if offered to all who could benefit, would be truly unsustainable.

As mentioned earlier, the state of Arizona recently attempted to hold down Medicaid costs by removing the most expensive types of transplants from coverage, including lungs and some liver and heart transplants, generating such intense outrage that the legislature reversed itself just a few months later. As reported in the *Wall Street Journal*, the decision was legal, but controversial because it was justified on the basis of questionable studies, and projected to save the state $4 million annually, while affecting a few dozen citizens each year (Bialik, 2010). This case nicely focuses the problem of technological proficiency: the development of new technologies can sometimes generate cost-effective improvements (kidney transplants), but also generates very expensive new capabilities. In advance of implementation, it is not generally possible to predict which outcome is more likely, and once implemented, even extremely expensive technologies become standard treatment.

Technology allows us, at very high costs, to perform life-saving feats. Once we have that technology, we then face the question of whether or not to provide it to those who need it. In cases when it is life-saving, refusing to provide it results in the patient's death.[2] But providing the treatment requires that resources be taken away from other people, who may not face immediately life-threatening conditions, but who are in serious need of those same resources; prenatal care, children with asthma, individuals with diabetes or high blood pressure, and so on. All of these individuals have some claim on the resources, provided they are available for public health. Diverting such huge amounts to a very small number (as happens in the case of organ transplantation) can leave large numbers of others in very bad shape, and can even result in an even larger number of deaths, though not deaths that will make headlines, as we noted earlier in discussing Nebraska's decision to cut prenatal care.

This problem is an entrenched one in health care, and it threatens to grow worse and worse in future years. Changes in technology, though they are often presented as an enhancement to autonomy, may sometimes force us to make choices where before we never needed to. The freedom to avoid having to choose is thus one that technology can diminish. We can see this in other areas besides transplant technology. Assisted reproduction has by now become such a standard part of contemporary life that couples who fail to produce a child within a few years of marriage are often asked directly what types of treatment they intend to pursue. The days when one could let nature take its course, and perhaps even welcome a life that might not involve procreation, if that was how things turned out, are no longer with us, however. In the contemporary world, the failure to procreate, especially for white

Western middle-class women, is generally treated as a disaster, and perhaps a moral failing, one that the woman in question must correct by any medical means necessary, even if that requires her to bankrupt herself, undergo painful and potentially dangerous procedures, and countless amounts of energy and stress (Gupta and Richters, 2008; McLeod and Ponesse, 2008). The technology has made it far harder for people to even admit that perhaps procreation is not all that high on their list of desired outcomes in the first place. Assisted reproduction offers for individuals the same issue that organ transplantation and other expensive technology offers for society as a whole—the forced choice between devoting extensive resources to these new technologies or being held responsible for the consequences of not using that technology.

As new treatments and procedures continue to develop, then, new demands on our resources will be made, and the presence of our background assumptions about the positive nature of technology will lead us, almost inexorably, to conclude that the resource must be used for these new treatments. Hence the dilemmas already noted in Chapter 3, as well as the consistent pressure on the aspects of health care that are not centrally affected by technology—the ever-growing pressure on nurses to provide care to too many, too sick patients; the migration of physicians to specializations rather than generalist positions; the general unwillingness to pay for such things as time and attention while tests and procedures are largely unquestioned.

The technological imperative drives a significant portion of public reasoning about the use and allocation of resources. This is both problematic and increasingly unsustainable. A second concern raised by the force of these new technologies is what I am calling the threat of dehumanization. (Clearly, this is not a neutral term). One place where this threat has been most clearly articulated is in the context of the new reproductive technologies.

Dehumanization of Central Human Relationships

Critics have argued that the new assisted reproduction technologies (ARTs) dehumanize fundamental relationships in at least three different ways. First, critics have charged that the new reproductive technologies change the very way children are perceived, turning them from 'begotten beings' into 'manufactured objects' in the memorable phrase coined by Oliver O'Donovan (O'Donovan, 1984; Ramsey, 1970). The argument is that technological interventions into reproduction cause us to see children as products of our manufacturing processes, rather than gifts from God. Most of the critics who have raised this concern have done so from a theological standpoint, and it was a very common argument in the early days of assisted reproduction. As the use of IVF and related technologies has become widespread, however, these concerns have tended to diminish.

A second, somewhat more nuanced criticism has taken the place of the 'manufactured children' critique as ARTs have become more broadly used. Critics have more recently charged that the new reproductive technologies disrupt the fundamental parent-child relationship by inserting so many possible new relationships into the mix: sperm, eggs, and embryos are all now available commercially. Parents can relatively easily (though at a cost) have a baby carried to term by a gestational surrogate mother. IVF permits embryos to be tested for genetic conditions prior to implantation. All of these various procedures and commercial relationships are destructive to the traditional connections between parent and child, according to various critics, because they change what should be a relationship of intimacy into one that is carried out by strangers (Kass, 1997).

Finally, a third set of critics have argued that ARTs dehumanize women (rather than children) by treating them as commercializable body parts. ARTs enable the sale of eggs, enable surrogacy, and function within an economic system that treats women's bodies as resources to be used for profit (Dickenson, 2001). Further, the marketing of ARTs demonstrates, according to these critics, an entrenched pronatalist attitude, one that consistently sends the message to women that if they fail to have children, they have failed at living a meaningful life (Corea et al., 1987; Hynes, 1991; Rowland, 1992). In both of these ways, by treating women as commercializable sources of gametes and gestational labor, and as existing for the sake of reproducing, ARTs, it is claimed, dehumanize women.[3]

All of these criticisms are worth taking seriously, particularly from an ethics of care. Because care ethics considers human relationships to be central to human life and to ethics, the charge that ARTs disrupt fundamental relationships and generate a tendency to see other humans as commodified or manufactured objects is clearly one worth taking seriously. At the same time, it is possible that some of the concerns critics raise are a bit sentimentalized and ahistorical (Brody, 2009). The fact that care theorists pay attention to basic human relationships need not entail that any claim that certain relationships will be changed by a new technology means that the new technology is morally problematic; the questions to ask are how the relationship is changed, and what that means for human lives overall.

So, what is it about the new technologies of assisted reproduction that might lead one to think in terms of the specific label of dehumanization? Humans exist and find their identity in networks of care. Because of this, they are irretrievably dependent on others for both their sense of self and their continued existence as a being of that kind. This is a descriptive fact about human existence, and the relationships that structure human lives can be either good ones or bad ones—the simple fact of relationality does not, itself, generate a positive evaluation of the relationships involved, though it does point to the central importance of relationships. When the language of dehumanization is invoked, it often signals a concern that fundamental relationships that shape human identity are being destroyed or corrupted, making those relationships function in ways that diminish the capacity for people to see themselves or others as fully human and valuable in the ways that human beings ought to be.

Consider concerns about all of the ARTs that are based on the commer-
cialization of reproductive 'parts and labor'—the practices that rely on buy-
ing and selling eggs, sperm, and embryos, and on arranging for gestational
surrogacy. All of these practices embody a deep contradiction regarding
procreation and what it signifies. On the one hand, those providing genetic
materials or gestational labor are expected to have no relationship with the
children who will result from the product they sell. Further, all of these practices treat the seller as an object of use. Surrogacy contracts, for example,
often require the surrogate to refrain from any number of activities (smok-
ing, drinking, rock climbing) while she gestates the baby, they often require
prenatal testing and a subsequent abortion if the child has certain genetic
defects, and they require her to agree to have no contact with either parents
or child after the contract is concluded and the child handed over (Steinbock, 1992). (Alternatively, in some cases the surrogacy contract is handled
entirely through attorneys to protect the anonymity of the purchasing parents.) The surrogate is treated as a commodity, as is the child; both must
meet certain standards of acceptability, and both are the sorts of things on
which one can set a dollar value (Rothschild, 2005; Shanley, 1995). Likewise, those who sell sperm or ova are expected to fill out forms in which
they 'sell themselves' by presenting the various aspects of their physical and
intellectual identity that make them desirable producers of genetic material.

Many of the new reproductive technologies are expressly designed to
make this sort of commodification easy and to distance the purchaser from
the seller while making the seller invisible. Those who will stand in a parenting relationship, on the other hand, are distanced in both physical and
relational ways from the process by which their child will be generated,
but are encouraged to think of the child they are paying for as truly theirs
because they are the ones providing money and making choices about which
donors or surrogates are acceptable. While the language of 'a child of one's
own' is used constantly to refer to the resulting child, those individuals to
whom the child is intimately related by biology or gestation are treated as
disconnected or invisible.

That invisibility, of course, indicates the problematic nature of the
relationship—when one wants the mother of one's children to 'just disappear,' there are problems in the relationship. It also indicates a desire to deny
the physical nature of the bonds that undergird some of the central relationships in human life. Parents think of a child, on this model, as theirs by right
because they paid for all or part of that child's genes or gestation; in the
case of surrogacy, however, the woman who spent nine months physically
carrying the child is erased from the picture altogether, while in the case of
gamete donation, the donor likewise disappears.

To the extent, then, that reproductive technologies embody the intent
to commodify parenting relationships while erasing the very people who
are vital participants in those relationships—to the extent that they not
only embody that intent, but obscure it as morally problematic by being

presented as miracle cures for infertility—they represent dehumanizing forces in the contemporary world. They both embody and make invisible a 'creeping capitalism' that turns relationships that should be exempt from economic calculus into marketplace transactions.

Now, it may be that my reader is prepared to accept these arguments for the dehumanizing effects of some of the new reproductive technologies, but may object that the problem is not the technology, but the context— procreation—which is, after all, a particularly fraught context with many ways that relationships can go wrong. In response to this objection, I would argue for two aspects of technology that do, I think, directly connect up with these concerns about dehumanization. The first has to do with the way that technology exacerbates the distance between parties in this case, and the concomitant erasure of the relevant relationships. The second is the issue of the way that technology in effect becomes a substitute for the relationship, and that can be seen in this case as well as other cases whereby technology, I will argue ahead, becomes a substitute for caring relationships in a wide range of medical contexts. But first, the issue of distance.

One of the ways that technology functions in many different aspects of the contemporary world is the way it allows action at a distance. Whether this is the capacity to call friends around the globe by Skype or the capacity to kill people thousands of miles away through drone strikes, technology functions to allow an agent to act in locations that are both physically and psychologically distant. In matters of procreation, then, technology does not just enable sperm purchasing; it allows the sperm to be purchased from an individual thousands of miles away, through networks that ensure anonymity. It also allows the embryos created with that sperm to be examined for genetic defects (or for sex selection) in a laboratory completely removed from the actual experiences of the individuals involved in trying to procreate. This is what technology does (not all that it does, of course): it makes the process whereby anonymous individuals can be in a procreative relationship with each other with no actual physical contact at all seem unproblematic and smooth. Psychologically, this makes the other person a non-entity—one is purchasing sperm, not generating a relationship with the sperm donor. But, as a matter of fact, the child will have a relationship (albeit an erased relationship) with the donor (who will be, like it or not, her father), and through the child, so will the child's other parents. Just as the distance at which we can kill in the modern world makes killing easier, the distance at which we can keep inconvenient procreative partners makes it easier to deny their reality and existence. Clearly, technology does not have to play this role—it can function in, fact, in ways that decrease distances— but when it plays the role of erasing other people in the relationship as people, it exacerbates already problematic relationships.

The second way that technology can function to dehumanize is in its tendency to be used as a substitute for caring relationships. Caring is hard emotional work, as anyone who has sustained a caring relationship over lengths of time knows. It becomes particularly difficult when the one cared for is undergoing a difficult time, or needs exceptional levels of support. In those contexts, it becomes very tempting to substitute technological fixes for actual caring. In the case of assisted reproduction, for example, one of the things that the technological wizardry helps to do is to avoid the need to think about why one wants children, and about how the desire for children functions in one's intimate relationships. Observers regularly note that undergoing infertility treatment generates stress for couples, and sometimes leads to divorce. It is probably worth asking why this is so, and what are the dynamics of the relationship (and their connection to procreation). I would expect to find as many stories, of course, as there are couples, but one theme does reappear over and over again in first-person accounts of infertility treatment, and that is the theme of a life that is empty of meaning without children (McQuillan et al., 2007; Olshansky, 1996; May, 1995).

When this language appears, it raises the question of what sorts of responses to a sense of meaninglessness are appropriate. There are, after all, many reasons why people experience a sense of meaninglessness or emptiness. Perhaps their life doesn't include many activities that provide a sense of meaningful engagement with the world, or perhaps most of their time is spent in isolation from the people and relationships that matter most to them. Rather than encouraging individuals to reflect on what changes to their lives might alleviate the sense of emptiness, however, the technology of assisted reproduction (and the associated economic structures) provide a ready-made answer (Sherwin, 1992). A feeling of emptiness, it is assumed, arises from not having a child. If one will just pay the necessary (and expensive) fees and undergo the various physical procedures, one will get a child, and a meaningful life will ensue. It is rare indeed for those providing assisted reproductive services to caution prospective parents that a child may not resolve their feelings of emptiness—and may, in fact, exacerbate them.

Further, there is an element of abdication of responsibility for finding one's own meaning in the whole process, as if one's life no longer needs to be questioned once procreation has happened. This displacement is particularly strong for women, given the extraordinarily powerful language of motherhood and the meaning of life as told to women. But as Simone de Beauvoir noted years ago, trying to achieve meaning or happiness through another's life is a problematic temptation for women. A mother is encouraged to "leave it to another to justify her life, when the only authentic course is to assume that duty herself" (Beauvoir, 1952, p. 551). While Beauvoir's language may a be a bit dated, the point she makes remains salient: trying to live one's life through another generates a whole host of ethical and existential problems. But this is not an issue that the contemporary world encourages people to think through. Instead, technology creates a world in which it is easy not to ask questions about what a meaningful life might actually look like, one in which that question has been answered by the whole system of assisted reproduction technology.

Technology, in this sense, directs our attention in a particular direction. Feel empty? We can solve that problem for you! And this is a dynamic seen over and over again in contemporary medicine. Feel unattractive and unfulfilled? We have gastric bypass procedures and plastic surgery that will solve that problem for you. Feel guilty that your elderly father is dying, and you've never had a good relationship with him? We can solve that by putting him through every possible medical procedure under the sun as he lies dying—we'll 'do everything' for him, so you don't have to examine those guilt feelings too closely. And, of course, it is not surprising that technology functions in this way in a consumerist society. After all, people spend money on technologies precisely because they do offer to solve our problems, not encourage us to work through the latest existential crisis. Perhaps there is no way to avoid this dynamic. Further, my analysis of the morally problematic nature of this dynamic is not an argument that it should be legally prohibited—the prohibition might be worse than the problem. But articulating and identifying how the dynamic works nonetheless seems worthwhile, if for no other reason than that it opens up the possibility of questions about when the technology might be worth rejecting in one's life, or when the technology might promise more than it can deliver. In writing this, I am struck by the similarities between the benefits technology offers and the way that having those available—while perhaps a good thing in itself, can generate other related problems because it allows us to avoid dealing with other, perhaps deeper, problems—is much like wealth.

Most of us, including the very wealthy, live with the deep conviction that if we just had more money, our lives would be better. But research on the wealthy indicates that not only does more wealth not increase happiness, it can actually diminish a sense of meaningfulness in life because it makes work unnecessary, and most people find work (with all its frustrations and annoyances) to be one central arena of meaning in life. Money also corrupts emotional relationships in predictable ways, and so on (Quoidbach et al., 2010). My argument here is that technology functions the same way. And, as in the case of wealth, the argument should not be seen as resulting in the conclusion that technology is a 'bad thing' and we should all go back to living off the land (or take vows of poverty, in the wealth case). Instead, the conclusion we should reach is that technology is a limited good, and so long as we treat it as such, it can provide many benefits. But the technological imperative tends to impel us to think of it as the ultimate good, so that we assume if some is good, more must be better. In pursuing this limited good, however, we may find that we are bypassing or losing altogether other, far more worthwhile, goods. The presence and pervasiveness of certain types of technology make the question of what we should pursue and why a hard question to even raise.

This is a theme to which I will return in Chapter 6 when thinking about end of life care, because it seems to me that the context of how we deliver end of life care is one of the areas where technology promises the most and delivers the least. But it is also a central feature of the problems of reproductive technologies because of their connection to procreation and to central human relationships. Like death, the technologization of birth and reproduction has the potential to change fundamental human relationships in ways that we may find problematic; but because technology is offered as the solution, it is hard to see that sometimes it may, itself, become the problem.

Unintended Consequences and the Technological Imperative

I have articulated two morally problematic aspects of technology—its unsustainable economic costs and its tendency to dehumanize essential human relationships. There is a third issue that needs to be considered, after which we will turn to the question of how best to respond to technology and keep it in its proper place. The third ethical problem with technology is that of unintended consequences, and it arises when those developing the technology are so focused on developing and using it that they pay no attention to other aspects of its implementation. All new technologies can be foreseen to produce results that are not the goal of the technology, but arise from it naturally just the same. One example is the way that the use of antibiotics is generating more and stronger antibiotic resistance in bacteria—many hospitals struggle with antibiotic-resistant strains of strep on a regular basis. Obviously, the researchers who developed antibiotics did not intend to generate these new strands of bacteria—but just as obviously, we cannot now ignore them.

It is common to assume that new technology, when it first becomes widely adopted, is largely risk free. So, my father remembers going to the shoe store as a child and sticking his foot in the x-ray machine to check the fit on his shoes. X-rays were wonderful things, and it wasn't until they had been in use for a while that people began to question whether all that radiation might be a bit of a problem. MRIs appear to be far safer than x-rays and CT scans, but a few animal studies have indicated that fetal MRIs correlate with certain teratogenic effects in mice. While the dangers appear relatively low, they justify caution, at least, in the extensive use of MRIs in early term pregnancies (Shin et al., 2011). That medical procedures may have unwanted side effects should no longer surprise anyone with any familiarity with medical technology. It is one of the reasons why any medical procedure must be fully explained to the patient to whom it is proposed, and why it should be the patient himself or herself who decides if the risks or known side effects are worth the benefit of the procedure. But it remains the case that it is frequently difficult to convince caregivers and patients alike of the importance of considering the costs of side effects. In recent years, debates over the cost/benefit ratios of frequent mammograms have demonstrated exactly this feature (Esserman and O'Kane, 2014; Woolf and Harris, 2012).

But there are also unintended side effects in terms of how technology changes the context within which we make decisions about medical procedures. The presence of new technological capacities shifts our understanding of responsibility for conditions that would have been attributed in the past to God, blind luck, or fate. For example, there is now a genetic test for one variant of Huntington's disease (HD). HD is a degenerative (and thoroughly horrible) genetic disease that begins in middle age, is inevitably fatal, and involves lengthy and unpleasant deterioration of neurological processes. Not all versions of HD appear to be straightforwardly genetic, but one version of it is, and the genetic sequences involved are dominant so that anyone with that particular genetic sequence can be predicted with 100% accuracy to be facing an unpleasant and untimely death from HD.

Now that the genetic test is available, two questions arise for members of families with a history of HD. The first question is whether family members should be tested for the genetic sequence. The testing (some argue) allows individuals to either stop worrying (if the test is negative) or make appropriate plans for the future (if the test is positive). Making appropriate plans was more difficult in the immediate past in the US, since insurance carriers considered a positive test to be indicative of a 'pre-existing condition' and so a reason to deny coverage to precisely the individuals who would need it, but that has changed with the passage of the ACA and other restrictions on insurance refusals. But other than purchasing insurance coverage and perhaps trying to experience some events a bit earlier in life rather than later, it isn't entirely clear what one can do to prepare for a progressive neurological disease that will occur at some unspecified point in late mid-life.

The second issue raised by the genetic test is the question of subjecting children to the risk of this disease. Some theorists argued that parents with a family history of HD should get tested themselves before having children; if they were to find out they carried the genetic sequence, they would have a moral duty, it was argued, to undergo IVF, and test any resultant embryos for the sequence (Savulescu, 2001). That way any children they brought into the world would not have to face such a horrendous fate themselves. As responsible parents, the argument went, they owed their children this extra step of protection.

In both of these cases—testing one's self, and testing potential children—there is a deep shift in the notion of what one is responsible for. Horrible diseases that have no cure and no prevention are almost the paradigm case of something for which one is not, and cannot be, responsible, yet the presence of a test moves this disease into the 'responsible' column, both for the individuals (who are thus confronted with having to choose whether or not to be tested) and for parents now accounted responsible if a child ends up with the same genes the parent has. (There is an underlying irony here, given our earlier discussion of the social pressure to procreate.) The presence of the test makes it impossible to choose to see one's self as not responsible; it shifts the playing field, so to speak, making the choice not to hold one's self responsible no longer an option.

The genetic test is, of course, marketed as increasing options for individuals; my argument is that in making some new options available, the very presence of the test closes off others that may be more choice-worthy from the perspective of the individuals involved, but they cannot rewrite history and put themselves back in a position of not having to choose. Technological changes thus bring in their wake changes in how people understand their lives and the choices they can (or should) choose from among. The re-framing of people's self-understanding represents a profound (and often ignored) unintended consequence of technological change.

Putting Technology in Its Place

In detailing these three problematic aspects of technological change in health care, I run the risk of sounding like a prophet of doom. This is unfortunate, as technology has brought enormous positive changes into human life right alongside the complexities it introduces. But the unfortunate fact is that the positives of technological change are clear, and widely advertised. It is important to note the unmentioned shadow side of technology, not because it is the only relevant factor, but because it tends to be ignored or repressed. Further, given the strength of what I have been calling the technological imperative—the pressure to adopt new technologies, and allow them to shape cultural and social structures—it is important to think not just about what positive technological change can bring, but also what it will take away from us, or in what ways it might diminish central aspects of caring relationships, or what impact the implementation of technology may have on other practices that we value (Winner, 1986).

From the perspective of an ethics of care, technological change represents both potential and peril. When technology is subordinated to human relationships of care, it can be wonderful thing (O'Keefe-McCarthy, 2009). When someone formerly dependent on weekly dialysis is finally able to receive a kidney and begin to participate in life's activities with renewed vigor, we see the real positives medical technology has to offer. But when technology defines care, it can become oppressive. A recent survey of palliative care specialists found that over half of the respondents had colleagues, patient's family members, or other professionals characterize palliative care treatments as euthanasia, murder, or killing (Goldstein et al., 2012). This tendency to accuse those offering palliative care of failing in their moral duties to patients represents the darker side of technology; the side that assumes that more is always better, that anything short of the maximum amount of treatment is failure, and that the only sort of care that medicine can offer is technological intervention.

Daniel Callahan, who has written extensively on the technological imperative, and to whose careful reasoning I am indebted in these pages, argues that we can never manage to 'tame the beloved beast' of technology until we begin to see ourselves and our use of medicine within the framework of a different set of values. While Callahan himself is not explicitly a care theorist, his analysis is one that fits well, in many ways, with an ethics of care, and is worth discussing in this context. He begins his proposed solution by arguing that our current medical model is a 'infinity model,' operating with built-in assumptions that, first, the benefits offered by technological interventions are infinite; second, that the resources available in medicine are infinite; and, third, that human life in infinitely extendable (Callahan, 2009, p. 146).

All of these assumptions need to be changed, he goes on to argue, because they are all both false and pernicious. So long as we assume that technology is an unmitigated and infinitely extendable good, we can never recognize that what it can offer is limited and comes with side effects that need to be acknowledged. So long as we assume that resources are unlimited we cannot recognize that even the goods that technology offers require trade-offs against other important goods. And so long as we assume that life is infinitely extendable, we will not be able to make decisions about what technological interventions are reasonable for different stages of the life span, and what are not.

What Callahan articulates is a set of revised values that begin with an assumption of finitude. We are fundamentally biological beings, with a limited and relatively predictable life span. When things go right in our lives, we start as infants, progress through childhood to adulthood, go through the process of aging, and then eventually die. Medical interventions that aim at a reasonable opportunity to progress through these stages clearly make sense. Medical interventions that aim at reversing the aging process altogether, or at staving off death for as long as possible, regardless of the cost in pain and suffering, or in health care dollars, make far less sense because they represent a failure to accept the basic condition of finitude that is part of the human condition.

Further, Callahan notes, we also need to recognize that the resources we can devote to medicine come from a limited pool, and demand sacrifices in other areas. Unlimited access to medicine for the elderly, particularly when coupled with the implicit assumption that we ought to aim to extend the life span indefinitely, will result in precisely the sort of spiraling health care costs that we currently face in the Medicare system in the US, costs that not only threaten many state budgets with bankruptcy, but also threaten other programs that we all value. Medical care for the elderly is of vital interest, but so are schools, police services, preservation of the environment, and roads. We recognize in other cases that limits need to be set in order to ensure a reasonable amount for other needs; the same limits need to be articulated for medical care.

Finally, we also need to recognize that the benefits of technology itself are limited in a number of ways. Health care professionals have gotten clearer and clearer in recent decades about the ways that technology can get in the way of care, rather than support care as it ought (Benner et al., 2011). Ethics committees over and over find themselves called in for consultations by caregivers who are trying to explain to families that the continued imposition of treatment on a loved one is not doing that loved one any good. Part of what makes it so difficult to intervene in such case is that the issue of whether to treat or not occurs against the background of the technological imperative, and, as I have argued, that produces background assumptions that the treatment (i.e., technology) will actually save the patient. Caregivers, having seen enough cases to know that technology doesn't always work, evaluate it as futile, and know it will cause serious harm.

How could this dynamic be changed? An ethics of care emphasizes the perspectival nature of relationships and interactions. Jeanette Pols argues that an adequate normative understanding of technology from the perspective of an ethics of care requires an empirical turn, integrating ethnographic empirical research with philosophical analysis. In particular, she advocates examining the relations between people in particular practices and the technologies that create part of the realities of those practices (Pols, 2015). She notes that when examining relationships, the questions one brings to the examination concerning what constitutes good care depends in large measure on the framings assumptions the researcher adopts.

This is a dynamic one can clearly see in the case of end of life care. From the perspective of caregivers, inside the context of medical practice, it is obvious that medical technology does not always help, and can sometimes do harm. But from the perspective of the patient and his or her family, this is not nearly so obvious. For people who do not work in the health care context, the main images of medicine are television shows that achieve miraculous results on a regular basis, news stories about the miracles of new medical technologies, and a reservoir of medical experiences whereby caregivers have provided care that solved the problem. Further, though there have been small steps toward involving patients in decisions about their own care, the bulk of medicine still operates with a model of mild paternalism, whereby a patient's right to know what all her or his options are is seen as an externally imposed restriction that gets in the way of good care. (This last is more true, in my experience, of physicians than of nurses.)

In the context of all of these forces, with the overwhelming force of the technological imperative running underneath it all, it is extremely difficult trying to convince a patient or a patient's family that although there are treatments available, they won't do any good and almost certainly will do harm. Treatments, by definition, help. Any chance seems better than death. And in the already fraught context of making decisions about the end of life, or about a loved one's death, emotions drive reactions far more than cold logic.

An ethics of care, faced with this situation, asks the theorist to take seriously the perspective of the families and patients involved, to respect the deep concern they generally feel toward their loved ones, and to think about the ways that their care and concern can be honored and protected while also encouraging them to recognize the limits and the drawbacks of technological responses. One of the most important responses is to keep the notion of care itself as the central focus of discussions of treatments.

Because medical professionals generally think in terms of what can be done to or for a patient, many discussions with the family begin (and often end) with a range of options to be offered. Part of addressing their needs, however, requires starting with listening to what the patients and their families see as their needs at the end of life (McDonagh et al., 2004) This allows caregivers to respond by exploring the various aspects of care that can be given, rather than listing the various technological maneuvers that can be done. To the extent that care can be the central focus of all discussions about next steps, and physicians and nurses can make sure that what is presented to the patient or to the family are options that make the care—not the technology—central, it may be possible to at least diminish the tendency to insist on treatment in order to offer care.

One very straightforward example of this, as many ethics committees have found, is to change the way questions about treatment are phrased. In the spirit of letting families make decisions, many health care systems will consult with decision-makers when a patient has reached the point of brain death, to ask when they want to turn off the ventilator and any other associated machines. What families often hear, however, is the question of when they want to kill their loved one. Not surprisingly, their reaction is rarely positive. Changing the question by prefacing it with an acknowledgment that they are not being asked to end their loved one's life makes a huge difference in how families respond to the issue. Explaining that their loved one is dead, then asking when they want the machines turned off, changes the way the question is heard, and often allows them to respond to the question that the caregivers need them to decide about.

Because patients and their families already face such difficult emotional decisions, and because they usually struggle to assimilate the information that is provided by caregivers, the burden needs to fall on caregivers to do what they can to avoid contributing to what Callahan has called the perspective of infinity. This sometimes requires speaking frankly about the fact that a patient is facing death, rather than always speaking as if the next treatment is going to cure her or his condition. This may require being clear about the side effects and suffering that any treatment will involve. Developing these traits of honesty and clear communication is a crucial component of addressing some of the issues the new medical technologies raise for us.

Conclusions

Technological innovation is unlikely to disappear from medical care anytime soon. The potential benefits for patients are too great, the potential for profit is also a powerful motive, and the assumptions that drive the technological imperative are clearly embedded in our reasoning and actions. The nature of the technology is likely to change. Just as the last 50 years have seen profound changes in what can be done and how it is done, it is likely that the health care of the future will be delivered in ways that are not possible now. Both genetic and nuclear medicine are in the experimental stages, and are likely to generate a range of new ways to respond to medical problems. The rise of computer-generated interfaces with human cognition, allowing for micro-surgery and related techniques, likewise seems guaranteed to fundamentally change many medical techniques.

But as much as the type of technology changes, the way it affects our lives and the basic caregiver/patient relationship is likely to continue to demonstrate the forces detailed in this chapter. Because technological changes represent the new and improved, the very presence of the technology will generate the assumption that it must be implemented. When the benefits are substantial, our faith in the technology will frequently blind us to the negatives it brings in its wake, whether increasing costs, medical side effects, or producing a problematic gap between caring professionals and patients needing care more than cure.

These are problems that cannot be resolved by more and newer technology. They are problems, instead, that connect up to who we are, what our lives do and should look like, and basic assumptions that we make about what matters in life. If we fail to think carefully about how technological changes affect caregiving, we may unwittingly allow the force of the technological imperative to sweep us into patterns of behavior and social structures that are not supportive of the sorts of care that medicine ought to provide. Whether we examine assisted reproductive technology, new genetic tests, improved imaging capacities, or organ transplantation, in all of these cases, the development of new technologies has put pressure on the delivery of health care, on patient responsibilities, and on our understanding of the parent/child relationships.

From the perspective of an ethics of care, responding to the challenges technology faces us with requires us to think about what does (and what does not) enable relationships of care. Because caring relationships require a high degree of personal connection, many technological responses to medical problems become barriers to engaged caring. We see this especially at the end of life, when over-medicalization of the dying process separates patients from family members, often renders them incapable of responding or communicating with others, and produces a process of dying marked primarily by intimacy with loudly whooshing machinery. This is a terrible way to die. We also saw how technological interactions at the beginning of life can alter the way that parents and children relate to each other.

But while an over-reliance on medical technology is problematic, a caring perspective also must recognize the ways that these technologies do speak to deep needs in human life. People are willing to pay huge amounts of money to fertility clinics because they often do feel that there are gaps in their lives, and multiple forces in our culture encourage people to turn to parenthood to fill those gaps. The technology serves a felt need, and a deeply felt need. The solution is not to denigrate any use of the technology whatsoever. Instead, it is incumbent on caring professionals to develop the capacity to maintain a slightly skeptical distance from the technology, recognizing the benefits it offers, but also recognizing the way that it can promise more than it really offers.

More than this, it is vital for us to articulate countervailing values—values of interconnectedness, relational wholeness, finitude, and caring—that can offer a set of alternatives to the technological imperative. Yes, providing organ transplants through Medicaid funding does save the lives of some individuals by the use of almost miraculous technology, but funding pre-natal care for vulnerable populations also saves lives, even when we don't know precisely which lives it may have saved. When we are faced with limited resources, we need people willing to point out that a choice to fund the most technologically advanced procedures may also be a choice to undercut other vital human relationships.

Ultimately, technological development cannot change basic facts about human lives. We were all born, we will all just as surely die, and we hope for meaningful lives with a reasonable modicum of contentment in between. Health care technology can serve human needs in wonderful and productive ways, but it needs to be kept subservient to human needs, rather than be allowed to define those needs for us. Unless we subordinate technological responses to care, the technological imperative may make real caring far more difficult for health care workers.

Notes

1 Terri Schiavo was a young woman who had been in a persistent vegetative state for a number of years. Her husband (also her legal guardian) wanted to remove her feeding tube, arguing that this represented her preferences. The Florida legislature intervened, passing legislation to allow the governor to prohibit the removal of feeding tubes in individual cases. The legislation was found unconstitutional. For one summary of the case, see Haberman, 2014.

2 The question of how to analyze issues of responsibility for someone's death in such cases is complicated. In specific cases, it is clear that someone who refuses to provide care can be held morally responsible, but those are cases in which there is a clear duty to treat. A general principle that anyone refusing to act in ways that could save another's life is thereby made responsible for their death, however, is untenable; even average-income US citizens have the economic capacity to donate sufficient money to famine relief to prevent some deaths, but that does not make them responsible for those deaths.

3 These are by no means the only criticisms of ARTs that have been made. Numerous critics, feminist and non-feminist alike, have been sharply critical of a range of reproductive techniques because of health risks to the children produced and the women who either donate eggs or gestate the child (Noah, 2003; Kaplan and Tong, 1994; Rowland, 1992; Lorber, 1992). Others have also criticized the use of ARTs in the context of inegalitarian economic and social power (Ryan, 2003; Purdy, 1996; Narayan, 1995). Other critics have argued that there is a fundamental bias against persons with disabilities embedded in ART practices (Rothschild, 2005; Coleman, 2002; Mahowald, 2000). This is not a definitive list, merely examples of the sorts of criticisms that have been made. The focus of my discussion in this chapter is specifically the charge that the use of ARTs dehumanizes the participants in one way or another, but this is certainly not the only reason why one might criticize such technologies.

5   Authority and Power in Medicine

Technology, knowledge, and money all have at least one thing in common: they are all sources of power. In earlier discussions of these various structures in medicine, the power each confers was largely taken for granted. But each of these structural aspects of medical practice exists within a highly structured system of power relationships, and without examining these relationships, we miss important features of how health care functions.

In earlier chapters, I have argued that there are at least a few basic principles for thinking about the shape of social structures from an ethics of care perspective. One is that care itself needs to be the focus of the structure; when the economic bottom line or technological innovation or large-scale statistics become the ultimate standard for medical treatment, patients suffer. A second principle is the need to face the limits within which medicine is practiced. We humans are not information-processing machines; we are human beings with limited information and limited processing skills, and we should structure the way knowledge is processed in medicine in light of what we know about human thinking. No economic system can be devised that will offer all the treatment anyone wants without incurring outrageous costs. Technology can be a wonderful thing, but every new treatment will also have unintended side effects that will need to be dealt with, and so on. We misconstrue what can and should be done in health care when we refuse to recognize the limits within which any system needs to work.

A third point that was especially salient in considering the way that insurance systems structure the delivery of health care also needs to be emphasized; structures that insulate those with power from having to see or deal with the consequences of their decisions exacerbate the tendency to benefit one's self at the expense of others. This effect of distancing is particularly apparent in the case of insurance carriers and patients; the number of states currently investigating health insurance companies for unfair practices is so large, in part, because the distance is so great between those making decisions about what to pay for and those who pay the price for treatments refused. So, issues of power have already been raised; this chapter will turn to them more specifically and situate them within the various power dynamics that function in contemporary medicine.

The Nature of Power and Authority in Highly Structured Social Contexts

Power is fundamentally a relational concept. To say that someone is powerful, or that a group has great power (or lacks power) only makes sense against a background that contains at least two relational concepts: a comparison with other, similarly situated people or groups, and a context within which certain capacities can be exercised. The first relation is the easiest to recognize. When I say that physicians, as a group, stand in a position of power (which is a true claim), I am making a claim about how they are situated relative to other, relevantly similar groups. In the context of health care, for example, we can compare the power relationships between nurses, technicians, janitors, patients, and physicians, and in this context, it is clear that physicians are a powerful group compared to the other groups in the relevant context.

But power is never absolute (except, perhaps, in a theological context), so the claim that physicians are powerful is not a claim that they have absolute power relative to others. Physicians may be more powerful than nurses in a health care context, but that does not imply that nurses have no power, and the same is certainly true of patients. Nor is a claim about physicians' power a claim about their being powerful in all contexts. On the battlefield, for example, physicians as a group are much more vulnerable and much less powerful than combatants. In countries where they do not have the organizational power of a group like the American Medical Association (AMA) behind them, they lack power in the political realm. Debates about the shifting nature of physician power have, in the past, focused on the proletarianization of physicians as their authority was undermined by HMOs and the corporatization of medical care (Mechanic, 1991), and more recent discussions about EBP also address the nature of the physician's authority (Upshur and Tracy, 2004). Statements about power, then, always require contextualization and should not be taken to imply any sort of absolute power differential.

The second aspect of power that needs to be kept in mind is that power functions in terms of specific capacities. Physicians may, as a group, be relatively powerful in a health care context, but the power they exercise is primarily power over events and policies within the specific context of the health care campus. One of the consistent frustrations physicians feel is the limitation on their power posed by the fact that patients go back to their homes and ignore the careful (or, occasionally, incomprehensible) instructions they have been given, leaving the physician feeling powerless and frustrated. Noncompliant patients, as they are termed, represent one of the limits to the power of health care professionals generally. Because power is not absolute, the fact that both physicians and nurses are more powerful in the health care context than are patients does not mean that they have absolute control over what patients do or choose, and though patients may have only limited power, they can exercise even that limited power in ways that frustrate the purposes of professionals immensely.

One of the mistakes we frequently make in thinking about power is to think that if one party in a relationship has it, others don't. As I hope is clear from the example in the previous paragraph, this is clearly not the case. Furthermore, power is not a resource like money that gets used up when it is exercised. Power functions in the opposite direction—to the extent that a person or group exercises power, they frequently gain more of it by exercising it. Among the reasons for this are the facts that power is relational and is constituted in part by social expectations and assumptions. Exercising power can put one in a position of greater authority, and so increases the power one is accorded by others to make decisions or to act.

Finally, one of the basic assumptions about power that structures feminist thought in general, and an ethics of care more specifically, is that while power imbalances are ubiquitous, and in some cases unavoidable, that never justifies systems that entrench arbitrary power (Held, 2006; Sherwin, 1992). Reorganizing hierarchical systems to permit more participatory power relationships, and structuring organizations so that power is exercised for the sake of those who are more vulnerable are basic moral values for an ethics of care.

While this very brief mention of some of the features of how power functions is not a complete analysis of the concept, it will do for the purposes of this chapter. I turn next to the question of how power is distributed in the health care context. And readers are reminded that in discussions of how power is distributed, I will be assuming both that this discussion is situated within the health care context, so discussions of relative possession of power should be understood as relative to others within the health care context. I also will be assuming that power is not absolute, so that in speaking, for example, of the physician's powerful role, I am not assuming that physicians have unlimited power, merely that among the various positions in health care, physicians stand in one of the more powerful positions (Flathman, 1982). It does not follow from this either that no one else has or can exercise power, nor that physicians' possession of power makes them somehow able to control everything that goes on in the health care context.

The power dynamics of the health care context are complex. Physicians, as mentioned, are one of the more powerful groups in that context, and their power flows from a number of sources. One of the first is knowledge. Physicians in many ways are seen as the final authorities on some of the most central issues of knowledge and determining the truth about things in the health care context. Their training consists of learning to diagnose—which in many ways means that they determine the nature of reality for many others in the health care system. They deliver the truth, and a truth about issues that are of potentially life-or-death consequence to patients. They decide what treatments will be provided or withheld, what body parts will or won't be cut off, or what tests will be ordered.

The power that physicians wield is complicated by other factors such as race and gender, however. Recent studies have noted that physicians who are women, for example, are treated with less deference than their male colleagues (Myers et al., 2018; Files et al., 2017). The medical context reflects the larger society of which it is a part in terms of its racial hierarchies, as well (Aberg et al., 2017; Bright et al., 2018), and these dynamics affect hierarchies of power in complicated ways. But they do not erase the structural power that physicians have compared to other medical professionals, and a significant part of this power is the capacity to establish what is or is not the case with regard to patients.

Compare this capacity to dictate the nature of reality with the situation of either nurses or patients. Both, of course, have control over some aspects of the health care situation. Patients control the information they provide, they can be willing or unwilling to go along with treatments, suspicious or trusting in their relationships with caregivers. They can be combative, or confused and wandering, or overly submissive. But when in an acute care setting, especially, their situation is a subordinate one. If they are too combative, caregivers will likely sedate them, regardless of their preferences. They will be expected to accept the diagnoses of their physicians and choose among the treatments offered. Patients who respond to a range of treatment options by asserting their right to choose a completely different option, whether alternative medicine, refusing treatment altogether, or some other modality, will certainly feel the disapproval and chill that accompany the refusal to submit to medical authority.

Nurses occupy an intermediate level within the health care hierarchy. Although they are professionals in their own right, the power they wield is very often one that relies relatively heavily on the authorization they receive from physicians. When a patient would prefer not to take a medication, the nurse frequently invokes the doctor: "Dr. X won't like it that you won't take this," or, "But it's Dr. Y's orders that you get this medication at this time." Nurses, for the most part, stand in a position between patient and physician; they have institutional power, rather than just the power over their own individual behavior that patients have, but a large measure of that power is to serve as proxy for physicians, rather than to function autonomously (Chambliss, 1996). Clearly, this situation is in flux; the rise of nurse practitioners functioning as independent medical professionals represents a clear shift in the power dynamics of medicine, and generates a concomitant set of legal and structural negotiations to determine how these new roles will be structured.

While it is relatively easy to identify the basic hierarchies of power in the health care setting, the relationships among those with varying degrees of power are always more complicated than any simple hierarchy would suggest. One of the paradoxes of power arises from the fact that the most dominant groups, those with the greatest access to power, have a deep dependence on those who seem to be powerless. (This is a point frequently made by theorists following Hegel's analysis of the master/slave relationship; see, for example, Mussett, 2006.) This is a particularly interesting feature of the health care context. While the role of patient is relatively powerless, it is, simultaneously, vital for the identities and sense of self of the caregivers who have so much more institutional power at their disposal. The result is a situation where the more powerful are psychologically dependent on the subordinate for their sense of self and identity (Mohrman, 1995). As a result, caregivers often feel tremendously vulnerable, in spite of the institutionally powerful positions they occupy.

Recalcitrant or suspicious or even just overly independent patients can pose a serious threat to the sense of self and of proper authority that caregivers feel. The situation varies, of course, from setting to setting, and is (at least in my experience) stronger in more traditional contexts, but there is an undertone of it in almost any health care setting. Patients who arrive having read all they can find out about what they think is their condition; patients who are suspicious of caregiver directives, or simply noncompliant in a variety of ways, generate a response that often seems out of proportion to the situation. But the reaction is not just to a single obnoxiously know-it-all patient, it is a reaction, instead, to an affront to the role of a physician (or, more rarely, a nurse) who is deposed from her or his position as one with authority to define reality (Brody, 1980). Instead of being an authority in such a case, the caregiver becomes one individual among others; instead of being powerful, she or he is demoted to a position that looks very much like that of an employee.

The vulnerability of professionals to this sense of being stripped of identity and authority is the source of some of the negative language caregivers use to speak about difficult or noncompliant patients (Meunier-Beillard et al., 2017; Tallman, 2018). When patients are aggressive or violent, of course, it makes sense for caregivers to react negatively, but the interesting cases are those when a patient is refusing treatment or questioning authority, but not in a particularly aggressive way. Those cases tend to generate intense negativity as well, even though it seems (to an outsider's eyes) to be not terribly problematic. The issue in these cases is one of a threat to the power hierarchy of medicine, not to specific caregivers, but the feeling of being threatened is real, nonetheless, generating very negative responses (Chambliss, 1996). As Tallman notes in her analysis of the power dynamics of noncompliance, "the whole concept of compliance is based on a power structure in which the doctor gives orders and the patient obeys (or doesn't)" (Tallman, 2018, p. 89). To the extent that a physician's identity is composed, at least in part, by the power and authority of the doctor's role, noncompliance poses a threat and generates very negative responses. As Tallman goes on to note, respect for patient agency and shared decision-making provides both an alternative method for dealing with noncompliance as well as defusing the physician's sense of frustration. Nor is medicine alone in this dynamic: professors facing students who question their authority act much the same way, and religious leaders faced with noncompliant church members as well. In the case of medicine, patient refusal to recognize the physician's authority and competence can intersect with racism, prompting patients to reject the authority of physicians from underrepresented groups, and continued experience of this dynamic can generate a crisis of identity for the physicians involved (Popper-Giveon and Keshet, 2018).

Human social institutions are complicated structures, dependent as much on shared understandings of social reality as on specific legal or economic structures. Maintaining them requires that most of those who participate in them accept the basic terms and structure of the institution, and act accordingly. The power structures of medicine, then, including the authority wielded by physicians, the middle-(wo)man position occupied by nurses, the relative powerlessness of auxiliary workers (secretarial workers, janitors, and the like) are a central part of how health care is delivered.

Power and Authority in Medicine

The power wielded by health care professionals is not arbitrary. The specialized knowledge physicians have and the extensive years of training in their field of specialization are legitimate sources of power, and justify much of the structure of health care delivery. The reasons most patients do trust physicians, and do rely on them for information, diagnosis, and treatment options, is precisely because they are highly trained professionals. Likewise, nurses are professionals with both schooling and practice-based knowledge of patient's conditions, responses, and outcomes. They are well-educated in the sorts of knowledge that most patients simply don't have, and a large part of the power they hold in the health care context arises from this specialized knowledge.

But knowledge is not the only source of power in health care. As Howard Brody notes in *The Healer's Power* (Brody, 1992), part of the physician's power resides in the hope and trust that patients place in their caregivers. Humans are essentially social beings, living within networks of trust and care. Especially when in the midst of a health crisis, we need the sense that those around us are powerful, knowledgeable, and have our best interests in mind. Patients who experience their caregivers as offering all of these have a far better experience, regardless of the outcome of their treatment, than those who feel they cannot trust their caregivers.

In addition to being repositories of trust and hope, health care workers also function as gatekeepers for a resource that people need. This aspect of health care was noted in Chapter 3; in the US, it is standard for any attempt to access treatment to be prefaced by a meeting with an administrative assistant who asks for insurance cards, identification, and various and sundry personal information. She (it is almost always a she) is not a health care professional in one sense, since her training is clearly not medical, but she is a central part of the health care experience for most patients, and can deny access if one's documents are not in order. Obviously, the situation is very different in countries with universal access.

Once in the system, it is primarily physicians and nurses who function as gatekeepers. Physicians can recommend tests and treatments, prescribe medications, and often run interference with recalcitrant insurance carriers. They control access to a wide range of health care options. Nurses, on the other hand, often represent the immediate gatekeepers for care—they are the ones who notice that pain medications aren't working and contact the attending physician to change a prescription or increase a dosage, and they are the ones who chart changes in condition (or lack of changes) and so make it possible to get this or that needed treatment. The gatekeeper role is an enormous source of power. When things go well, playing this role consolidates the health care professional's standing as a respected and trusted authority figure.

So, among the sources of the caregiver's power we find specialized knowledge and expertise, trust and hope, and the gatekeeper's role. All of these sources of power are interwoven in complex ways with the economic and institutional/legal structures of contemporary health care. Hospital administrators, for example, about whom I've said little in these pages, can make the roles that health care professionals play either difficult or smooth. Legal regulations on (for example) the number of hours residents can work at any one stretch affect the ways that physicians understand their relationship to patients, and the sort of knowledge they can bring to their role. Recent studies of the limits on residents' hours have found that while shortening their hours improves the residents' quality of life, it also leaves them without the intense connection to an individual case that used to mark residential training. It was common in former times for a resident to stay right through a whole course of treatment with a patient; with shorter hours, residents now hand off patients to others, raising concerns about continuity of care (Coverdill et al., 2010).

As in all cases of relationships marked by imbalances of power (as most relationships are), caregiver/patient relationships can generate a whole host of ethical concerns. In turning to these concerns next, I want to make clear that I do not advocate some utopian vision of health care without power imbalances. (Such a vision is both unattainable and undesirable. It is unattainable, since medical professionals should know more than their patients. It is undesirable because if we either pretend to have absolute equality of power or strive for that result, we are likely to make tremendously bad policy choices along the way.) Nor do I blame health care workers for all of the things that can go wrong in the relationship between caregiver and patient: patients are moral agents themselves and are to blame for a whole host of problematic relationship issues. But in spite of the fact that much of the time, medical relationships are beneficial and work very well for both caregiver and patient, the power imbalances and structure of the relationships lends itself to specific types of ethical problems, and to that I turn next.

Ethical Issues Generated by Power Imbalances

As mentioned earlier, the hierarchy and resulting power imbalance that structure the health care relationship are not something that can be gotten rid of. Medical professionals really do have more knowledge than patients, they do control patient access to treatment and care, and neither of these issues is likely to change any time soon. Various structural changes in health care in recent decades have shifted some aspects of this structure, of course, making information more readily available to patients outside private discourse with one's physician, imposing strict requirements of informed consent on treatment regimes, and the like. These changes represent changes in the relative power of patient and caregiver, but they do not equalize power.

Whenever a relationship is marked by large disparities in power, there are a number of standard ways in which it can go wrong. In this section, I will enumerate some of these standard corruptions of power, and consider how they function in the context of health care. As mentioned earlier, I do not think these characterize every health care interaction; on the contrary, I think most interactions are much smoother than this. But the ethical problems arise frequently enough, and are sufficiently characteristic of the health context that they deserve attention.

On the caregiver's side of the equation, the three dominant sources of power all offer opportunity for problems in the relationship. I'll begin with knowledge and expertise. I've noted already that for some physicians, patients who do their own research are seen as problems. This phenomenon, which is at least anecdotally common, indicates one way that the power that knowledge confers can become problematic. When an individual's status as 'expert' becomes an end in itself, and they are more concerned about being the most knowledgeable person in the room than being a person with useful expertise, the power of knowledge has shifted from existing primarily for the good of the patient to serving to consolidate the physician's authority. The knowledge then serves as a status marker for the individual who has it, not primarily as something that serves the needs of others. It is a bit unfair to pick on physicians alone here, since anyone whose job involves a good deal of difficult or less-well-known expertise can fall prey to this same vice, but the problem it identifies is real.

Standing in a position of expertise also puts one at risk of claiming more knowledge than one actually has, in order to avoid being shown up as less knowledgeable. This is especially tempting to residents, early in their education, who really don't yet know all they should, but are nonetheless interacting with patients as physicians. It is tempting in cases of this sort to bluff, and it would be unrealistic to expect that residents would never resort to such techniques. It is a good deal less innocent when long-time practitioners do it. In both cases, however, the shift to EBP noted in Chapter 2 offers a useful antidote to the temptation, since a physician trained to check out the literature on the case will be far more comfortable with saying that more research may be needed. This is a temptation to which clinical judgment models make one more prone.

Knowledge and expertise also, however, generate a paradoxical temptation when a caregiver knows more than he or she believes that he or she can tell the patient. Both nurses and physicians who function as part of a team will understand this issue: when a patient asks directly for information, either about the expertise of another physician, or questions about a diagnosis or a prescribed treatment, the other caregivers can find themselves in a difficult situation. If the patient's concerns are legitimate, admitting that fact can put caregivers in a very difficult spot with their colleague. But failing to respond to the patient's concerns honestly represents a failure of care, and a concomitant failure in the caregiver's duty to put the best interests of the patient first. It is an especially difficult situation for nurses who can suffer real and serious repercussions from a physician who feels his or her actions have been questioned by someone who has no right to challenge the physician's authority.

In all of these cases, however, the misuse of power arises, in part, from the fact that the knowledge that the professional has is turned into a source of status and power for himself or herself, rather than being used for the benefit of the patient. Ideally, of course, the two are not in conflict, but work together. When things go right, the professional's expertise functions for the benefit of the patient, and because it so functions, the professional also receives respect and acknowledgment, not as the direct goal of her or his action, but as the rightful response to expertise. But given human psychology, it is all too easy for the respect and acknowledgment to become the goal of power, rather than a byproduct, and in those cases, the power of knowledge is used against the patient, rather than for the patient.

This is a dynamic that recurs in the case of the other sources of power in medicine, as well. Consider the power that physicians wield in terms of representing hope and comfort to the patient. Again, the power is legitimate, but should primarily be turned toward generating the most positive environment for cure that is possible. It can be tempting, however, for physicians to use this power in ways that are not to the benefit of the patients. When, for example, patients are encouraged to join clinical trials that are not terribly likely to offer benefits to them directly, this power can prove very effective at motivating patients, but to their potential detriment.

The gatekeeper role, likewise, represents a source of power that can be misused when caregivers use the threat of lack of access to force compliance or extract obedience from patients. There is, of course, a very fine line here between legitimate refusals to offer treatment the caregiver believes to be ineffective or futile (which may or may not result in a patient changing his or her behavior or choices) and using the threat of withholding treatment precisely for the purpose of manipulating patient behavior. Given that most of the time, caregivers are legitimately focused on the best interests of the patient, most deliberations about what can or cannot be offered are good-faith exercises. But a patient who challenges the status quo, especially a noncompliant one, does represent a tempting case for using power in threatening ways (Playle and Keeley, 1998).

When we note that caregivers can use their power inappropriately, especially when that power is used to protect their own self-identity or protect their prerogatives or manipulate another, we should also note that patients, though having less power than professionals in the health care context, nonetheless have source of control and authority, and are as prone to misuse them as anyone else in the situation. The constant threat of lawsuits that physicians in the US find themselves subject to is one way that patient power can function pathologically.

Recourse to the law is a necessary part of the current situation in the US. There are some physicians who should not be practicing, and patients can find their lives ruined (or worse, ended) by an incompetent surgery or a negligently misdiagnosed condition. In these cases, patients should have some recourse, and the only one available in the US is a legal one. It might be far wiser for the medical system as a whole to set up a less adversarial system for resolving disputes about treatment, but so long as lawsuits are the only option for patients, they will be legitimate in certain cases. But the power that the threat of a lawsuit represents can be, and at times is, misused. Patients can use threats to try to force physicians to respond in any number of different ways, and the threat of monetary losses is not really the worst of the threat. For most physicians, the real power of a lawsuit is the attack on one's sense of self as a competent and caring professional. Fear of lawsuits, in fact, is cited as one of the major reasons that physicians leave the practice of obstetrics, a field in which the sense of competence and caring is particularly salient (DeVries et al., 2009). Lawsuits by necessity represent the professional as incompetent or negligent, and for a professional this is felt as an assault on their personal integrity.

Likewise, patients can use their limited ability to provide or withhold information as a source of power. In many cases, this is especially tempting to patients who are suspicious already of the medical establishment, who tend to self-medicate extensively with alternative medicines (herbs, extracts, enzymes, and vitamins) and who often refuse to pass this information on to caregivers (Becker, 1985). The situation this sets up, whereby caregivers cannot accurately diagnose or treat because of the other substances a patient is taking, while the patient refuses to divulge what exactly is being taken, is rarely a positive one. When, in addition, the physician feels threatened by the patient's lack of trust and respect, and resorts to some of the manipulative uses of power just mentioned, things can go very wrong very quickly (McCullough, 1999).

This particular dynamic represents a real danger when racial and ethnic differences enter the picture. Racism casts a long shadow in the US medical context, and racial disparities in a variety of areas, from pain control to treatment of heart disease, remain a concern. In this context, patients who fear that they are being offered second-class treatment due to their race or ethnicity are prone to mistrust their caregivers, while caregivers may respond out of unconscious bias to their patients. This exacerbates the dynamic of mistrust and misuses of power described earlier.

Nurses, like every other population in the health care context, also can be prone to certain typical misuses of power. One of the interesting phenomena in health care is the tendency for a small subset of nurses to use their mid-range position in the power hierarchy to bully those they have power over, much like mid-level bureaucrats the world over tend to bully the civilians with whom they come into contact (Lewis, 2006; Rocker, 2008; Dellasega, 2009). While the numbers of nurses who bully is small, their influence is tremendously pernicious to both the care team as a whole and to patient care.

Because of the in-between character of the nurse's position, there is also a temptation to play off one side against the other in any perceived power plays. Sometimes nurses encourage patients' suspicions of competent physicians, in order to shift patient loyalty to the nursing staff. Other nurses are tempted to side with and protect physicians inappropriately, and to see their role as disciplining patients who fail to show sufficient respect. Again, because power always brings with it the potential for misuse, and because nurses play such a vital role in mediating so many relationships in the health care context, it is clear that the power they wield can be misused in a number of ways.

Care Analyses of Power

One of the issues that can be noted in all of the cases of misuse of power mentioned in the preceding section is that the power of the health care setting should be directed toward the well-being of the patients who present for diagnosis, healing, or reprieve from pain. When the sense of self of the professional or the protection of one sub-group or the patient's sense of control become the central focus of the use of power, things go badly. When, on the other hand, power functions to serve the internal goods of medicine, it is used properly.

From the perspective of an ethics of care, this is what would be expected. Care flourishes in relationships when power is not focused on protecting the powerful, but instead functions to support and nourish the vulnerable. Care theorists have argued that the mothering or parenting relationship is particularly significant from a moral point of view because it provides insight into how relationships of care ought to function (Held, 1993), especially when there are marked imbalances of power, and this discussion bears out their arguments. Unlike a social contract account of ethics that operates with an assumption that moral agents are equal, rational, and roughly equal in power, care theory recognizes that many moral relationships are characterized by imbalances of power.

But even though this basic principle is clear, it is less clear how to structure the relationships, and the social structures within which they function, to ensure as much as possible that this is how power functions. Obviously, no social structure can ensure that power is never misused. There will always be individuals who abuse positions of power and exploit the vulnerable, which is why legal remedies and criminal courts will never go out of business. The question, then, is not whether one can set up a system in which no abuse of power ever occurs; the question is how to set up systems in which such abuses are kept to a bare minimum, for most caregivers it is relatively straightforward and unproblematic that power will be used for its proper ends, and the system itself does not foster abuses.

More than this, systems of health care delivery need to keep in mind the various ways that imbalances of power influence what viewpoints are considered authoritative, and which voices are silenced. Reflexive systems that allow feedback from those enmeshed in the system allow for these imbalances to be confronted or revised, at least in some cases (Gilson, 2014; Walker, 2009). So, the proper structure of authority and power in health care needs clear systems of accountability and responsibility that allow themselves to be challenged.

Joan Tronto addresses exactly this issue in her discussion of informed consent (Tronto, 2009). While standard discussions of informed consent treat it as a requirement developed to protect patient autonomy, Tronto argues that it is better understood as a grant of authority. If informed consent is supposed to be protecting patient autonomy, she points out, it fails miserably. Many patients in the health care system lack the capacity either to understand or to evaluate the information they are given, and the fact that patients overwhelmingly accept whatever treatment is offered under the guise of informed consent in these conditions suggests that what is going on in this context is not authentic autonomous decision-making as it is understood in standard philosophical accounts of autonomy.

The problem here, Tronto argues, is that standard accounts that equate consent with autonomy lack a clear sense of the place of power in medical decision-making. Informed consent is intended to provide some protection for patients against abuses of power on the part of caregivers, and given the imbalance in power between these two groups, the intention is an important one. But so long as consent is seen as acquiescence to the power of the professionals in the health care setting, the imbalance in power is left unaddressed.

Tronto advocates a change in the way that consent is understood, from consent-as-autonomy to consent-as-authority (p. 189), arguing that so conceived, consent becomes the creation of a new relationship, one in which the professional gains the authority to act, but also the responsibility to exercise that authority in ways that fit well with the purpose of the consent—namely, to achieve the goals that the patient aims at, and to do this in a way that acknowledges the ongoing relationship between caregiver and patient. "[A] grant of authority is an act of trust," she writes: "the assumption made by the grantor is that the person entrusted will act in ways that are consistent with the reason one consented and granted authority in the first place" (p. 191). While the autonomy framework for consent focuses on the patient's rights and violation thereof, the authorization framework focuses on the caregiver's responsibility for carrying out the patient's intentions, and protecting the patient's interests. It highlights the fiduciary nature of the caregiver's role, and locates the relationship in the context of the broader practice of health care more generally.

The discussion in earlier chapters has noted some of the ways that the structures of health care can facilitate or hamper caregiving, and these offer a starting point for thinking about well-ordered structures of care. Consider the earlier discussion of knowledge, and its structure as a matter of evidence-based knowledge in the contemporary health care context. EPB does offer some very important structural support for the proper use of power in what I earlier called its democratization of knowledge. Whereas physicians working with a clinical judgment model of knowledge are more likely to feel that knowledgeable patients threaten their status as expert professional, physicians used to literature searches and relying on others' research are less likely to be threatened by patients who do their own research (Rodwin, 2001). In an EPB system, that is what is expected, and any source of (reasonably reliable) evidence is worthy of consideration.

Further, the democratization of power built into an evidence-based system affects the relationships between caregivers, allowing a more holistic understanding of knowledge-based authority that allows a range of medical professionals to speak as experts in their field (Gabbay and le May, 2011). Given the extensive evidence that shared decision-making teams produce better outcomes for patients, systems of knowledge creation that allow all caregivers to contribute to the care of patients is both morally and practically a better system (Grumbach and Bodenheimer, 2004; Litaker et al., 2003; Hearn and Higginson, 1998). Likewise, a new emphasis on collaborative decision-making, and on structures that facilitate patient understanding and participation in decisions about care, offers a far better paradigm for shared power than top-down authority ever can (Higgs et al., 2008; Politi and Street, 2010). The benefits of sharing authority produce measurable improvements in patient outcomes (Higgins, 1999).

In addition to this positive, EBP also builds in a sense of fallibility. Working, as it does, with percentages and hypotheses, it does not require the clinician to demonstrate an intuitive diagnostic omniscience, but instead portrays diagnosis as a series of hypotheses needing to be investigated (Timmermans and Angell, 2001). Again, this structure is one that is conducive to working with the patient as a partner, rather than framing the caregiver/patient relationship as one of authority and submission. Diagnoses are more likely to be framed in terms of, "Well, it's likely that you have condition X, so let's start there. If you don't respond, then there are other possibilities." On the clinical judgment model, this sort of admission of probability and exploration would be indicative of a lack of authoritative knowledge; on an EBP model, it represents the paradigm of medical epistemic practice.

On the other hand, EBP also incorporates some structures that do not always support the proper use of power. Its heavy reliance on statistical evidence and large-scale studies can make it easier for clinicians to view patients as statistics—to treat them 'by the numbers,' as the phrase goes—rather than taking the time to focus on the individual in all his or her particularity. Because the paradigm of knowledge is one of aggregated numbers, it trains clinicians to think in terms of generalities, and while good clinicians will resist this pressure, it will require resistance on their part; the social structure itself pushes in the opposite direction.

This pressure to see patients as statistical entities, interchangeable and undifferentiated, is exacerbated in the contemporary world by the pressures to hold down medical costs. As I noted in both Chapter 3 and Chapter 4, there are powerful forces in contemporary medicine driving up the costs of delivering care, while the economic resources available cannot possibly keep pace. And because many payments for services are provided in the US by insurers, there is even more pressure to follow clinical practice guidelines automatically, rather than think through what a particular patient might need. This can be particularly problematic in the case of elderly patients with co-morbidities, which can have serious health consequences, and, ironically, result in over-prescribing of medications (Boyd et al., 2005). Further, because medical care tends to be defined in terms of technological prowess, the non-technological aspects of medical care (time spent talking with a patient, for example) are not reimbursed, while tests and procedures are. The result is a system that puts enormous pressure on clinicians to see large numbers of patients for very short periods of time, treating them as largely substitutable entities who need a quick scan, a series of diagnostic tests (the more standardized, the better) and then a prescription. Good physicians, again, will resist this pressure as much as possible, but my focus in this book is not on whether some physicians manage to be caring regardless of the circumstances; my focus is on whether the system itself is conducive to good caring. My contention is that these intersecting factors are not conducive to good care, and while the physicians who manage to deliver it anyway deserve our respect and commendation, it would be better to restructure the aspects of the system that make it so hard for them to do what they do.

The power dynamics that structure the situation under which nurses provide care are more complex in many ways than those between physician and patient. Nurses are in a position of power over patients, especially when the patient is particularly fragile or needing intensive care, but they do not have the same level of institutional power that physicians are awarded in contemporary Western culture. Patients are more likely to argue with them or refuse to comply with basic procedures, and because they have so much more contact with patients (at least in an acute care setting), they can face exhausting and draining challenges to their authority on a regular basis. Further, because nurses are less powerful relative to physicians, they also find themselves dealing with the frustrations that accompany that relationship, facing physicians who are sloppy in their directives, unwilling to respond when questions are asked, or simply abusive because they can get away with it.

In the worst cases, this can create a toxic brew wherein nurses bear the brunt of frustrations from both patients and physicians. Burnout is tremendously high among nurses, and this may be one of the reasons (Kraus et al., 2011; Garrosa et al., 2011). At the same time, paying attention to how these dynamics function can allow the health care context to be structured so that the situation does not become so toxic. Team approaches to patient care, for example, that diminish the power disparity between physicians and nurses, allowing all members of the health care team to work together to provide good patient care, have been demonstrated to diminish burnout (Heponiem et al., 2012). When the interactions between nurses and physicians are ones of mutual respect and teamwork, not surprisingly, there is far less of the abuse of power that can characterize physician attitudes toward nurses. Likewise, when a health care system provides both clear information to patients about what is (and what is not) acceptable behavior, and protects nurses and other professionals from mistreatment and disrespect, it can expect an improvement in nurses' experience and attitudes. Treating patients with respect is a moral requirement; allowing them to act in ways that are abusive and demeaning to the medical staff is not.

An ethics of care does not always advocate responding to those cared for in ways that they prefer. In parenting relationships, for example, part of being a caring parent is precisely not giving children everything they demand, but instead providing clear and consistent boundaries within which their development can go on in a healthy way. In caregiver/patient relationships, likewise, a caring response to an abusive or violent patient is not one of permissiveness. It shows no respect for an individual to treat them as if they have no control over their behavior, and I take it that respect for another is a central aspect of care. Part of care, then, requires a response that sees the capacity for responsible action in the other and acts to encourage behavior that makes a healthy caregiver/patient relationship possible.

In normal cases, caregivers should be able to expect that a patient's responses and behavior will be that of a responsible adult. Obviously, the situation changes when caring for children, adults with serious mental illness, and cases when a medical condition affects a patient's capacity to process information or control his or her emotions. When the patient does not have any of these extenuating conditions, it is reasonable for caregivers to expect the patient to control her or his responses, behave responsibly, and treat caregivers with civility. Deciding when to demand decent behavior and what methods of enforcing that demand are all themselves decisions that are subject to moral scrutiny, of course, but the basic point is that expectations for basic comportment are not, in and of themselves, morally unacceptable or paternalistic. Quite the contrary; having reasonable expectations for patient behavior is a mark of treating the patient as an adult rather than as an uncontrollable and unreasoning child.

Most of the issues of power mentioned so far are relatively obvious in a health care context. There are, however, some less obvious aspects of power that are worth scrutiny both because they can be so much a part of how health care systems function that they are largely invisible, or because they tend to be treated as somehow outside or tangential to the health care system, in spite of being crucial components. Unspoken assumptions about the nature of health care fall into the first category; insurance systems fall into the second.

I'll begin with the first. Sociologists have demonstrated on numerous occasions that both physicians and nurses tend to hold a slightly different set of values than the average patient. This is not surprising, since the system whereby physicians and nurses are educated and the context within which they work is a relatively specialized system. So, there is both self-selection into the health care field, and then further character formation that goes on as a result of spending long hours in a very specific community of health care workers. Some of the significant features of the way physicians and nurses think include a tendency to value independence and the ability to be self-sufficient more than non-health care workers. The result is a relatively consistent finding of differences between health care workers and patients in assessments of quality of life (Sprangers and Aronson, 1992). Health care workers also tend to define 'effective medical care' more strongly in terms of chance of cure than do patients and their families, particularly when considering cases of disability. The disjunct between caregiver assessments of expected happiness or quality of life, and that actually reported by clients or their families in the case of disabilities, has given rise to the so-called disability paradox. When the condition that caregivers believe should be corrected is not permanent, however, the frustrations caregivers can experience in such cases can be quite severe.

That different demographic groups have different assumptions and expectations is not in and of itself a problem, but it can become problematic when the group which stands in a more powerful position does not recognize that differences exist. Health care workers are regularly frustrated by noncompliant patients because in their professional role, they spend nearly every waking moment focused on protecting or restoring health and functionality to their patients. When the patients themselves are (or seem) lackadaisical about their own health or when they engage in practices that are clearly contributing to loss of function, health care workers think they are at best irresponsible, and at worst self-destructive. Consider, for example, the common case of a diabetic who does not control her blood sugar well, does not work hard on keeping her feet clean and healthy, and is regularly presenting with infections that don't heal because of the poor circulation that accompanies poorly controlled diabetes.

From the standpoint of caregivers, our hypothetical patient fails on any number of levels. She doesn't keep her diabetes under control, the results of that failure produce serious complications for the circulation in her extremities, and she also fails to address those problems—and if she can't be bothered (it seems), then all the time and energy caregivers devote to her care are just wasted. It is tempting to write her off as a drain on the whole system. From the patient's perspective, of course, things may look quite different. She may be faced with multiple demands on her time and energy. If she is holding down two different low-wage jobs, and is desperate not to lose what little insurance she currently has, trying to parent one teenager and three grandchildren whose parents aren't able to give them consistent care, doing this in a neighborhood with little access to healthy food and no good public transportation, she may let issues of preventive health care fall by the way. It isn't that she's stupid—she knows she'll pay the price for it, and regrets that. But too many issues in her life are too urgent, and she can only do so much in one day. Careful food preparation after a 12-hour shift with nothing to eat in the house is simply not going to happen. Lengthy and careful cleaning and examination of her feet are likewise low on the priority list, especially when the few hours she has off work involve talking to a teacher about a child's disciplinary problems in school, trying to get the landlord to fix the hot water heater, and dealing with a neighbor in an abusive relationship.

Both the perspective of the health care workers (people need to take responsibility for their own health issues) and of the patient (that will have to wait—I only have time and energy for these other issues right now) have their place. But in the health care setting, it is the health care worker's perspective that defines reality. Patients who fail to follow instructions are considered irresponsible, and often shamed, subtly or not so subtly. In the health care setting, health is what matters. The entire structure of the system is built on that premise. So, within that context, those who fail to take what seem to be simple and obvious steps to preserve health are seen by caregivers (and often see themselves) as irrational and irresponsible.

In a similar way, those who refuse treatment or question medical advice are also framed as problems, since they challenge both the authority of the caregivers and the basic values that infuse the health care system. And so long as patients function solely as individuals, the power dynamics within medicine ensure that their challenges or failures are attributed to them as individuals, framing them as the problem, rather than any systemic issue.

On the other hand, when patients band together, they can often generate systemic change that can be quite effective. Groups such as Death with Dignity, Not Dead Yet, La Leche League, and various disease-specific support groups have all managed to be relatively effective in generating changes in medical practice and in the assumptions made about treatment and patient choices. So long as patients function as individuals, the lack of power they have undercuts any attempt at changing the system; even demands for specific modifications of a quite modest sort are met with such a weight of resistance that it becomes almost futile. When individual women who did not want their labor and delivery to be treated as a medicalized event argued for alternative treatment in the 1960s, they were largely ignored, but when groups began agitating for the possibility of Lamaze and other natural birth methods, hospitals slowly began to change.

This has been particularly evidence in the case of end of life care. During the 1970s and 1980s, medical technology for sustaining life grew far more effective, and the assumption in the health care setting was that everything that could be done for every patient should be done. The result was that the percentages of people who died in the hospital setting reached the highest levels ever, the resources spent on end of life care soared, and the dying process for individuals was turned into a grueling, over-medicalized and lengthy sequence (Lavi, 2007). Individual patients or the families of patients who tried to intervene and prevent some of the excesses of this approach were treated as problems: the families were suspected of 'wanting Granny dead,' while the individuals were simply dismissed as mentally ill.

When Death with Dignity was formed, however, and began pursuing a broad range of strategies, from providing instruction manuals on how to commit suicide to making the legal right to refuse treatment more widely known, and the like, it changed the way end of life care refusals were seen (Hillyard and Dombrink, 2001). Health care workers began to distinguish between treatment aimed at curing specific conditions and palliative care that aimed at responding to pain and discomfort when no treatments could provide cures. It became commonplace for health care workers to distinguish treatment when recovery was to be expected from treatment that did little more than extend the dying process. Legislatures passed laws requiring patients to be informed of their rights at the end of life, including their right to elect DNR orders and to select family members to make medical decisions for them.

Two things are striking about the way that end of life care has changed since the 1980s. The first is the availability of hospice care for terminal patients; hospice is a wonderful thing, and it is unlikely it would ever have become available if it weren't for groups such as Death with Dignity agitating for the right to commit suicide (Siebold, 1992). There is an important lesson for how power is structured in this dynamic. Because patients refused to accept the treatment that the health care system was offering, the system changed. But it took a long time, in part because the power hierarchy of medicine made it very difficult for patients' voices to be heard and because the entrenched authority of physicians, coupled with a focus on curative techniques rather than care, made it difficult to recognize the harms that medicine can cause. This is a classic example of the way that entrenched power structures can undermine the central goals of a practice such as medicine. It is also a valuable reminder that the response of those on the receiving end of care is a crucial aspect of evaluating what constitutes good care.

The second striking change in medical care at the end of life is the way that what originally was the standard dynamic (individuals agitating for less treatment, hospitals insisting on doing everything) has flipped so that today most ethics committees see exactly the opposite dynamic—patients (or more usually, their families) demanding more treatment while caregivers try to argue them into less treatment and more palliative care. There are interesting racial and ethnic aspects to this dynamic, with African-American families being more likely to want life-sustaining treatment and much less likely to want physician assisted death under any circumstances (Krakauer et al., 2002). The differences are closely connected with levels of trust that patients and their families feel toward caregivers and the health care system in general. Addressing the issue of trust will require a continued process of working to generate structures of care that allow all patients to feel that their voices are heard.

Faced with the obviously miserable and extended dying process that was (rightly) being criticized by groups such as Death with Dignity, health care systems had to become somewhat more self-reflective about the way that patients were being treated in their last days, and to face the fact that many health care workers themselves were horrified at what they were doing to their patients. Once that process started, the move to a hospice-based system and the shift from forcing treatment to withholding treatment were both natural next steps.

So, while patients are (as individuals) relatively powerless in the context of health care, as a group—and particularly as a vocal group—they can have a significant effect on the way that treatment decisions get made. This would be the final point to keep in mind in thinking about the way power functions in the health care context: power accrues to groups rather than individuals, for the most part, and to the extent that any group can function as a unit in a setting such as health care, to that extent they gain a voice and the power to argue for their own position. But so long as they remain individualized, their voice will lack the volume needed to gain recognition.

This sets us up for the next chapter, a discussion of the ends of medicine with specific reference to the issue we have concluded with here—end of life care. End of life care brings together all of the themes that this book has focused on, from the overuse of technology to the economic structure of health care delivery. And it should not be surprising that the way we die reflects so many of the tensions in the way we live today.

Conclusions

Health care is an enormously powerful societal structure. In economic terms, it commands a huge percentage of the gross domestic product (GDP) and provides jobs and professional status to huge numbers of highly skilled workers. In terms of the resources devoted to medical technology, it is one of the most important areas of new technological developments in the contemporary world, and in its speed and scope of implementation of new technology, it rivals almost any other area of modern life. In terms of knowledge and expertise, medicine is situated at the very powerful juncture of theory and practice: as a science-based practice, it has the epistemic prestige accorded fields such as physics and chemistry, while as a practical field, it offers the resources of that knowledge in concrete and effective treatments for some of the most central threats to human life.

For the most part, the power that medicine wields is exercised for the benefit of the patients who need its services. The vast majority of medical practitioners—physicians, nurses, technicians, and therapists—put the well-being of their patients first and foremost. But any practice that commands as much social power as medicine does will be susceptible to abuses of that power, and there are aspects of the way medicine is structured that sometimes facilitate specific sorts of abuses. Economic structures that penalize practitioners who spend time with patients, for example, or that create a distance between individuals with the power to deny treatment and the patients to whom treatment is denied, both generate forces that make it difficult to truly care for patients. Good physicians and exemplary nurses may resist these pressures, but as structural forces, they undercut the moral response that caregivers should offer to patients.

Much of the focus in traditional ethical analysis of medicine has been on individual choices and decisions, but in this chapter, especially, we can see how the power structures of medicine function in ways that channel and constrain individual choices. Without this broader perspective on the ways that social structures determine what options are even available, and what conditions structure the decisions that individuals make, we miss the range of ethical issues facing contemporary medicine.

From the perspective of care ethics, there are specific problematic issues in contemporary medical practices. Physicians and nurses who serve as gatekeepers for patient care need to recognize the various ways that their power can be used for both positive and negative ends. They can enable needed care, but that power also allows them to use threats of withholding treatment to force patient compliance even when the patient has legitimate reasons for choosing otherwise. The hierarchical structures of medical care likewise are open to abuse, as are the many resources of technology. What is important to recognize in so many of these cases is that the occasional abuses are not necessarily simply a matter of bad choices by individuals; there are often structural features of medicine that make it hard not to fall into these patterns of behavior. Change, then, should not be thought of as a matter of rejecting technology or denying that hierarchies of power exist in medicine; responding to problematic structures requires acknowledgment of the structural effects and a willingness to address that side of the ways that care is organized and delivered.

Structural changes of this sort are usually slow to be implemented, and rarely occur without unanticipated side effects. Both of these can be seen in the many ways that end of life care has changed in the past 30 years in American medicine—and to that we now turn.

6 Conclusions

Care, the Ends of Medicine, and the End of Life

As I write this, a friend sits in a hospital room, watching over her baby. He was born far too early, at a stage health care workers call 'micro-pree-mie.' Babies at this stage are so small they need microscopic sizes of every-thing: intravenous lines, diapers, needles, and monitor equipment. He was born so early that it will be more than a month before he can even tolerate being touched and stroked: at this point, parents and visitors are asked to speak very quietly, keep the lights dim (or off), and keep skin contact to a minimum.

It is a terrifying matter to be making decisions for a baby like this. There are no guarantees that any medical procedure will help, no guarantees of survival, and no way of knowing whether he will have serious develop-mental problems or not. And in the context of all this uncertainty, parents are asked to make choices about the lives of their babies. My hope for my friend is that these decisions will not turn out to have been decisions about end of life care, but rather decisions about procedures that will protect this little one's life and health, but at this point, neither of us knows what the outcome will be.

I begin with this scenario as a reminder that decisions about end of life care rarely fit the stereotype offered in medical ethics classes. With a back-ground picture of informed consent and patients' rights running through our minds, we are likely to envision decisions about life and death matters to be made by the patients themselves, after being fully informed of the risks and benefits of any given treatment. Our legal codes, in fact, assume a pic-ture much like this, and then try to fit the complexities of actual cases into that rather uncomfortable straitjacket. But as often as not, end of life care is provided to patients who are incapable of making decisions. Many decisions are made without knowing whether or not they constitute end of life care—it is only as the situation unfolds that it is discovered that the condition is so serious, or the complicating factors so, well, complicated, that these might be the last days or weeks of someone's life.

Patient autonomy, likewise, never works out the way the courts assume, with a clear-minded rational adult making choices based on her central life values (O'Neill, 1984). Patients are confused, caregivers cannot always communicate information clearly, time is not always available for careful deliberation about options. Family members may have strong opinions about what sorts of treatments are appropriate, and their opinions may not be congruent with what the patient wants, or would have wanted. Families are messy, emotional, complicated things, and end of life decisions exacerbate the emotional complications. Further, outcomes are uncertain, and no one knows whether a given procedure will provide relief or healing, or instead generate complications that will make the last months of the patient's life completely miserable. Miscommunication abounds, between caregivers and family members, between patient and loved ones, between well-meaning friends and individuals struggling to come to terms with their own mortality.

The complexities of personal relationships are magnified, in turn, by the complicated structure of contemporary medicine. As noted in earlier chapters, the delivery of contemporary health care is structured economically (the best care money can buy!) and technologically (do everything!) in ways that almost require maximization. Some of the deepest conflicts in end of life care occur when patients or their families disagree with caregivers over the proper use of technology at the end of life, or the economic limitations on providing medical treatment. The end of life is existentially fraught, a time of spiritual and subjective intensity (Spiro et al., 1996). It can hardly be otherwise. Religious and social authorities intervene, offer advice, make laws, and legislate options. Individuals at the end of life are enmeshed in all sorts of social relationships and connections, some of their own choosing, but many unchosen and some unwanted. Readers needing an example of the latter might think of the case of Terri Schiavo and how it played out on the national stage as an example of just how complicated these relationships can get. But the complications that make providing good end of life care do not stop there.

End of life care generates deep conflicts between some of the central goals of medicine. What makes medicine the sort of practice that it is are the ends it pursues: its orientation toward preserving and maintaining health, its capacity to prevent or cure illness and injury, its alleviation of pain, and its role in preventing premature death and prolonging life (Hanson and Callahan, 1999). But in end of life care, these goals run into inevitable conflict. Preventing death may require imposing pain, not alleviating it. Procedures aimed at restoring health may unwittingly shorten life when complications set in, or when a patient's body is just too weak to heal. Since all of these goals are central to medicine's identity, the conflicts they generate in end of life care have no easy resolutions.

Throughout this book, I have relied on an ethics of care to think through the issues raised by various social structures in medicine. In this chapter, care ethics provides a vantage point for bringing the various parts of those discussions together. No ethical theory can make the end of life uncomplicated or easy, but an ethics of care does offer a perspective from which we can see why some of the complications arise, what can be done to mitigate them, and how we might approach the various issues in ways that provide a more caring, less conflicted context for dying patients.

Care, Finitude, and Modern Medicine

The first aspect of care ethics that offers an important set of considerations for end of life care is its recognition of finitude (Sevenhuisjen, 2003; Groenhout, 2004). Both caregivers and those who receive care are finite, embodied people. Caregivers have limited resources, and usually need to care for more than one individual. The resources they can draw on are limited, and there are multiple demands on those resources, as well. This is obvious in individual cases. The most loving parents in the world can only devote a finite amount of time and energy and family resources to any one family member. The attempt to provide unlimited care to any one produces stark inequalities in how others are treated, and can generate an unhealthy sense of entitlement in the individual getting all the attention. Part of caring well involves setting limits on how much can be demanded, ensuring a reasonable level of fairness in distribution of time, attention, and money, and helping all the members of the family see each other's needs and entitlements, as well as their own.

The same need to recognize limits and the need for sharing recurs at the level of social practices such as medicine. Reasonable limits need to be set when determining what is demanded of caregivers, particularly those providing direct hands-on care. No individual or group can be allowed to demand unfair amounts of care, nor should more resources than they even want be forced on the dying. As a matter of abstract principle, this is easy to see; the problem comes when attempting to work out policies and general practices in the concrete that reflect these general principles.

As I noted in Chapter 4, the development of new technological capacities is not merely a neutral matter of providing resources that can be used freely in whatever way individuals think is best. Instead, the very presence of technology changes the structure of human life; it changes definitions and values, and it changes the meaning of the choices people make. In the case of end of life care, the very presence of intensive care units, for example, make it necessary to decide whether or not to pursue aggressive care at the end of life. That decision, in turn, creates a whole cascade of other issues, from the amount of money spent on end of life care to questions about whether family and friends can (or should) be present during the patient's last days to deliberations about whether withdrawing treatment can ever be morally acceptable once it has started.

The perspective of care provides a way of thinking about these issues that prioritizes care and caring relationships. More specifically, the automatic assumption that true caring will require that caregivers utilize any and all technological interventions possible gets the relationship between caring and technological intervention exactly backwards. Much of the medical technology available for end of life care actually diminishes a patient's capacity to remain in contact with loved ones. Spending the last days (or months) of one's life in an intensive care unit, attached to multiple machines and monitors, with all the necessary limits on visitation that a sensitive environment such as the ICU requires, makes remaining in contact tremendously difficult. Further, the environment of an ICU is hardly conducive to comfortable interpersonal interactions—one can hardly imagine a less relaxed or homey environment (Walling et al., 2010). This is not a criticism of ICUs, which are designed for a very specific purpose (delivering very exacting medical support) and perform that task very well. The point, instead, is that if the focus in end of life care is on protecting interpersonal relationships, caregivers will not automatically assume that more treatments and interventions are always better.

Clearly, the hospice movement offers exactly the sort of alternative that is preferable here. But far too many patients find themselves in the ICU in spite of not wanting to end their lives in that environment, and in spite of trying to make their wishes clear. Part of the reason for that is that medical technology does not exist on its own, but is integrated into the complex authority structures of contemporary medicine. For many elderly patients, the location where they spend their final years is a skilled care facility, where they may have talked through their choices about end of life care and perhaps even requested that no extreme measure be taken at the end of life. But when they need medical treatment that goes beyond what the facility can offer, they are transferred to a hospital, and their earlier decisions may not transfer with them (Lynn and Goldstein, 2003).

In-hospital care is acute care. The entire system is set up to provide the highest level of medical procedures possible. Even patients with very limited capacity to understand are allowed to consent to any procedures the hospital can offer; it is only when someone wants to refuse treatment that their capacity to consent may be called into question. More than this, legal requirements structure the hospital setting so that the default mode is treatment. Failure to treat leaves the hospital open to lawsuits, either on the basis of failure to perform with due care, or on the basis of discrimination against age or disability. Treatment decisions are made by specialists in the various conditions a patient may have, not by the sorts of more generalist, holistic practitioners often working in a skilled care facility. As the patient enters the hospital setting, she finds herself in a different country with different rules, and the rules are all directed toward using whatever resources are available to actively address conditions.

Again, the focus in the hospital setting makes sense, given that the vast majority of those who enter its doors are there to be cured or at least stabilized, and many of them need that care with an urgency that requires immediate and (relatively) automatic treatment. But when the whole structure of an institution is geared toward active treatment, the institution may not serve the needs of particular categories of patients, particularly those whose greatest need is for comfort care rather than aggressive treatment. For the fragile elderly, particularly those with advanced dementia, the care offered in a skilled nursing facility may, in fact, produce outcomes that are as positive as an acute care setting, and without the burdens of a disorienting move, dislocation from established relationships, and intrusive procedures (Gozalo et al., 2011). Use of the emergency room, in particular, tends to come into direct conflict with the goals of a more hospice-style approach to treatment (Lambda and Quest, 2010); again, not a surprising result given the very different goals of these two systems.

One of the most striking differences between a nursing home, hospice facility, or home-based care system and an acute care setting is precisely the different attitude each exhibits toward the use of medical technology. In a nursing home or a hospice setting, technological interventions are treated as something to be approached carefully, mindful of the side effects, negative potential, and dangers of use. In the acute care setting, technological intervention is the default mode, and any failure to provide it requires an explanation. One of the lessons we might learn from care theory is that acute care settings might learn from long-term care on this matter a bit, and recognize that the pressure to utilize technological interventions can undermine attempts to provide good care. There are certain specific times when a focus on care can remind caregivers of this possibility: when technology requires that family members and others 'get out of the way' so that medical personnel can do their job (not always inappropriate, but always worth thinking about), or when technology is functioning as a substitute for care. We often see this latter case when estranged family members insist on excessive treatment to assuage a sense of lost opportunity for loving relationships.

In the American context, economic incentives interact with the availability of technology in the acute care setting to generate even more pressure to intervene. A patient who occupies space in an acute care setting, but on whom no tests are performed and no procedures done, represents a net economic loss for the system as a whole. Although people speak of fee for service as an economic structure, it is less service than tests and technology that generate revenue. True service work involves attention and time, but neither constitutes a billable expense. In what was probably the most shameful politicization of the Affordable Care Act, in fact, one of the few true 'services' to be covered, namely end of life counseling, was dubbed a 'death panel' and eventually completely eliminated from the Act. What we have, then, is a fee for procedure system, coupled with a perceived need for defensive medicine to protect caregivers from lawsuits.

Again, beginning from the vantage of care helps put the economic structures into perspective. Patients, their families, and their caregivers are justifiably skeptical about money-saving systems proposed by insurers and government bureaucracies, because they suspect that cutting costs is an end in itself for both. In Chapter 3, I argued that when those who are making decisions about what to pay for are distanced from those who suffer the consequences, the structure of the relationship makes it much more likely that patients will be treated badly. At the same time, requiring decisions about properly allocating resources to be made by dying patients and their caregivers is not a workable solution, either. A patient facing her own death ought not be asked to decide which treatments are so expensive that she should forego them, nor should her family be asked to put a dollar value on her life. In actual practice, physicians often find themselves making allocation decisions, often without adequate support or a clear sense of the best way to make such decisions (Hurst et al., 2005), and this type of 'bedside rationing' is hardly ideal, either.

All of these options are problematic because they place the responsibility for making general economic decisions about funding medical care in the hands of individuals who are either too close to the situation or too distanced in the wrong ways. It might be tempting to think that something like John Rawls' committee of fully informed rational agents, all committed to living with their decisions once the policies are drawn up, could resolve the problem of what policies to have (Rawls, 1999). Unfortunately, theoretical committees, such as the members of Rawls' committee who reason behind the veil of ignorance, tend to reach the conclusions of the individual imaging what such a committee would conclude. Worse, since they are all, by definition, identical with regard to their reasoning structures and information, there is no real deliberation involved in such a procedure at all (Benhabib, 1992).

When real committees grapple with developing guidelines for medical expenditures, the policies they develop are rarely accepted by those to whom they are intended to apply. In some cases, committees that made decisions that seemed eminently the deliverances of common sense were seen by the public at large as deeply problematic. Consider, for example, the committee charged with deciding who would receive dialysis when it first became available. Given the extremely limited number of people they could accept into the program, the committee chose to allocate dialysis to the individuals who (among other characteristics) seemed the most deserving, either because they had children or were productive members of society. Because of this they were criticized harshly for 'playing God' (and nicknamed the Seattle God Committee), and many current guidelines for medical decision-making try to exclude what have come to be called social worth factors in their decision-making (Jonsen, 2007; Lockwood, 1988). Further, their processes and policies for making decisions were almost immediately overturned by media pressure.

Another example of a failed attempt to generate fair policies by committee occurred in the state of Oregon. The goal of the process was to rank-order treatments in order to provide the greatest number of citizens with the greatest possible access to Medicaid. Focus groups and town meetings were used to decide what resources were available and what treatments should be covered, and the result was a widening of accessibility of Medicaid coverage to ensure that most of the state's citizens would have access to basic health care. But in order to generate that level of coverage, some of the most expensive procedures were not covered, including liver transplants. Within months of the plan going into effect, a young boy needing a liver transplant was denied coverage and made a cause celebré in the local media. The demand for coverage made the expansion of Medicaid unsustainable, and Oregon went back to covering only a small portion of citizens (Jacobs et al., 1999; Kitzhaber, 1993).

While philosophers like to imagine that there are rational ways to develop systems of resource allocation, in the real world, such decisions will inevitably involve political machinations, media exposes, and all the other messy features of life in a relatively free society. That doesn't mean that there aren't better and worse responses to allocation questions, just that any system developed will be subject to all of these pressures—and to that extent will be irrational and sub-optimal. That said, however, it is worth noting that attempts to develop spending guidelines and principles for coverage that are based on concern to provide care occupy a very different moral terrain than do spending guidelines driven by a concern to improve profit structures. Whether requirements for basic health care coverage are set by government policy or by special committee or by citizen focus groups, in any case the criterion by which decisions are made needs to be that of care. This requires, then, that policy groups be clear that profitability (of insurance carriers, of pharmaceutical or equipment manufacturers, of physician's groups) is not their main concern. At the same time, however, there needs to be some structure of accountability; decision-makers ought not be cut off from those about whom they make decisions.

Recognizing that these are the features necessary to generate a reasonable policy for decisions about spending decisions allows us to also recognize better and worse systems for making decisions about end of life care. For example, decisions that are left to the discretion of a for-profit insurance company are likely to be problematic in any number of cases, and to generate skepticism even when they are legitimately made on the basis of medical criteria. Decisions made by physicians at the bedside will offer a high degree of arbitrariness, since different physicians have very different opinions about when care is futile, decisions made by political appointees will reflect political commitments, and so on. To the extent that any of these decision-makers are disconnected from the effects of their decisions, so that patients and families have no way to appeal decisions or negotiate, the system will be problematic.

As Nel Noddings and other theorists have noted from early on, care cannot be defined purely in terms of what one person does to or for another. For an action or a policy to exhibit care requires (for the most part, and under normal circumstances) a feedback loop that allows those receiving care to respond and acknowledge or challenge the nature of the action.

Institutional care also requires a transparency to third parties, an openness to scrutiny that ensures the fairness and healthiness of decisions and policies (Noddings, 1984, p. 69). If structures of transparency and feedback are not built into decision-making processes, we can assess them as failing one important test provided by care.

Advocating structures of transparency and feedback is hardly innovative, of course. Almost every business feels compelled to ask for feedback or evaluation after even minor transactions, and many health care systems make sure that there is some sort of follow-up with every patient after discharge in order to ensure quality control. This is, overall, a good thing. But the short term follow-up generally fails to elicit deeper reflection on the more general questions about whether the care provided met the needs of patient and family, whether earlier (or later) discussion about hospice would have been better, whether the use of technology and treatment protocols was worth the expense and disruption for the patient, and what advice the family might offer to others going through a similar process. Informed families offer an important resource for thinking about what sorts of care are most important for end of life care, and also what sorts of barriers to care the acute care setting (or the hospice setting) might generate. Recent movements to provide quiet hours in hospitals during the nighttime, for example (Gardner et al., 2009), were generated by following up with patients about what factors in a hospital stay were most problematic.

Something as simple as the opportunity to sleep quietly through the night is often far more important for a patient's experience than many of the expensive tests used to ensure 'high-quality care.' Giving the patients and their families a voice in the process does not necessarily generate increased costs, and may lower them in cases where the type of care that is most needed is basic consideration, comfort, and support, as is so often the case in end of life care. And in all of this, acknowledging the limits of resources helps to remind both caregivers and patients and their families that the resources for providing medical care are not unlimited but need to be used wisely, guided by a concern for providing the best care possible for dying patients.

But in recommending this sort of feedback loop, we run up against another way in which acknowledging finitude and limitations is tremendously difficult in a health care setting. Health care professionals have prestige and authority based on their expert knowledge of various aspects of medicine or health care. In the context of medical institutions, their authority is enormous, as discussed in Chapter 5. Recognition of the authority of the patient and the patient's family, as is necessary to produce truly valuable feedback loops, requires a concomitant acceptance of the limits of physician authority and knowledge—and this is a very difficult thing to recognize, particularly for physicians themselves. When one's identity is generated, in part, by expertise and widely respected knowledge of a complex and difficult practice, it can be very hard to simultaneously recognize the limits of one's knowledge and authority.

This difficulty may be mitigated, to some extent, by the move to implement EBP. As discussed in Chapter 2, one of the signal strengths of an account of medical knowledge that places the primary authority in experimental results and research rather than the individual's clinical judgment is an increased acceptance of multiple sources of knowledge. Likewise, a culture of respect for various types of authority, which some health care systems work to foster, can make this sort of recognition possible, as well.

Accepting limitations and the finite nature of both resources and care available can produce a health care system that deal with end of life cases more realistically and in a way that is more caring. But clearly, more is needed in developing systems of end of life care that both meet patient needs and work within sustainable systems of care provision. One of the reasons for the astronomical level of expenditures at the end of life comes from the way that the ends or goals of medicine structure the provision of end of life care.

End of Life Care and the Ends of Medicine

In *After Virtue*, Alastair MacIntyre analyzes complex practices such as the practice of medicine, and argues that the identity of a practice is determined by the internal goals of the practice (MacIntyre, 1984). A practice such as medicine necessarily has a wide range of goals; standard health care systems in the US have goals that range from making a profit to becoming an area's primary heart care system to expressing religious ideals through providing medical care to improving patient satisfaction. MacIntyre distinguishes among these various goals by pointing out that some of them are external, while others are internal. Internal goals are those that are central to the identity and nature of the practice itself. Health would not be health care at all if it no longer aimed at providing care that maintains and protects health, for example. External goals are ones that may be important for all sorts of reasons, but which are not part of the very meaning of the practice. Making a profit, for example, may be required to keep a particular health care system in existence, but it is not what makes it a health care system, and other systems can be health care systems while being organized as not for profit. Profits, then, are external goals, while acting to protect health is an internal, identity-constituting goal.

Distinguishing between internal and external goals is important for two reasons. The first is a practical reason; because internal goals determine the very identity of a practice, they need to be kept central, not subordinated to external goals. A for-profit health care system obviously needs to remain fiscally sound, but if making money becomes its main goal, and health care is subordinated to profit-making, then the practice is corrupted in predictable and morally problematic ways. Medicine has long recognized that the health and well-being of the patient have to remain at the heart of medical care, and for most caregivers, that central focus defines their role in society.

One of the benefits of examining medicine through the perspective of an ethics of care, in fact, as noted in Chapter 4, is that it puts economic factors into perspective. There are a number of different ways to organize the economic structures of medicine, but all of them need to be evaluated by their impact on the provision of care. Economic systems that generate too great a barrier to receiving basic standard care are simply inappropriate for the practice of medicine (as I argued in that chapter that a completely free market with only fee-for-service payment structures would be). Because medicine is not simply a business, but is a practice organized and identified by the internal goals of providing care, protecting health, mitigating injuries and curing diseases, any economic structures appropriate to that practice will need to further the actual goals of medicine.

The second reason why identifying internal goals is important is an analytic one. Conflicts in how medicine is practiced often arise from conflicts between internal goals that then become intractable because the goals are each (or all) centrally related to the identity of medicine. Unless the conflicts among goals are thought through, the practical conflicts are irresolvable. End of life care is a classic example of precisely this phenomenon.

Mark Hanson and Daniel Callahan have identified four goals or ends of medicine, which they argue are not culturally relative but universally accepted as central and internal to the nature of medicine. The four they identify are: (1) health promotion and maintenance, and the prevention of disease and injury; (2) relief of pain and suffering; (3) care and cure of people with maladies, and care for those who cannot be cured; and (4) the avoidance of death and pursuit of a peaceful death (Hanson and Callahan, 1999, p. xi). End of life care sits uneasily in the midst of these four because at the end of life, the various goals prescribe different responses.

When an individual is dying, promoting health and preventing disease become difficult or even impossible. Relief of pain and suffering, while possible, can come into conflict with curing maladies. A patient with an advanced case of cancer that has metastasized and caused multiple organ failure can either have her pain treated or her cancer cured, but the care team will find that these two goals pull in different directions. Avoiding death may no longer be possible at a certain point; accepting death may be required for psychological health in many cases, but will come into conflict with the goal of improving and protecting physical health. End of life care, then, identifies areas where the normally coordinated ends of medicine pull apart and generate tension.

The social structures examined so far in this book intersect in important ways with the goals of medicine, and an ethics of care provides a helpful perspective for seeing those intersections. Patients and families receiving end of life care face difficult decisions about when to pursue treatment and when to forego it, when to treat pain aggressively and when to try to tolerate pain for the sake of either treatment or simply a clearer mind. They often face clashes between psychological health and physical health, especially when treating their condition with chemotherapy, for example, will produce so much pain and nausea that spending time with family becomes agony. Add to these issues the fear of death and generalized existential anxiety as well as difficulty understanding complex medical terminology and even the meaning of probabilities, and the decision patients are faced with are simply daunting.

In years past, the response to all of this was for physicians to take on responsibility for decision-making, often without even telling patients that they had other options. The medical ethics literature from years past has extensive discussions of whether physicians should tell the truth about their condition to dying patients, with lengthy arguments offered in defense of the claim that the patients would experience so much fear and anxiety at receiving the news that it was a physician's duty to spare them by withholding the information.[1] Surveys of patients regularly indicated that they preferred to know the truth, but physicians maintained the right to decide whether or not they could handle it. The paternalism exhibited in these discussions was clearly generated by a deep concern for the well-being of the patients, but it co-existed alongside an inability to recognize that while truthful disclosure could be painful, the long-term problems caused by a lack of truth were worse. Dying patients need to know their status, even though it is a painful thing to hear, because they need to have an honest assessment of their condition to make sensible decisions about whether or not to continue painful or debilitating treatments, about how to deal with family issues, about whether or not to get a will updated, and all sorts of other issues.

Because physicians focus on physical health and illness, their assessment of whether or not patients should be informed of their condition tended to be framed in terms of that aspect of a patient, as well as on how the psychological effect of getting bad news would affect physical health. Patients, on the other hand, while concerned about physical health and illness, placed that aspect of their lives within the broader context of their family relationships, business responsibilities, and many other factors. Their knowledge of their own affairs, not surprisingly, was far broader and more nuanced than their physician's knowledge could possibly be, and their capacity for making decisions for themselves thus better than their physician's capacity could possibly be.

From an ethics of care perspective, none of this is surprising. From early days, care ethics has emphasized the need for ethics to take a particularistic perspective on ethical decision-making, rather than try to generate absolute, general, universal rules. It is easy, of course, to overstate this point, and turn deontological or utilitarian theories into simple minded rule-generators, or care ethics into an overly simplified situational ethics. The truth of the matter is that traditional Western ethical theories generally have the capacity to acknowledge particular circumstances, while an ethics of care can acknowledge the importance and relevance of general rules and principles. Having noted this, however, the universal/particular distinction is nonetheless one of the salient differences between a care approach and a deontological approach to ethical issues.

As mentioned in several of the earlier chapters, care ethics mandates a focus on the specific relationships that shape and support people's lives. In the case of end of life care, it is clear that these relationships are of preeminent importance, perhaps more important than they might be at almost any other juncture in a person's life. Care ethics demands that we pay attention to how these relationships function, to the ways that the social structures of medicine (economics, technology, knowledge, power, and the like) affect them, and the ways in which they can be strengthened and protected in a health care context. I have already argued that many of the structures of medicine tend to undermine or complicate interpersonal relationships, and this is particularly evident in certain aspects of end of life care. The technological prowess medicine has developed is a wonderful thing, but it can be enormously destructive of personal relationships at the end of life. Because the presence and widespread use of technological interventions is assumed to be central to providing the best possible medical care, it is prioritized even when it disrupts the human relationships that may be far more important during a patient's last days and hours.

Hospice care, obviously, has been designed to offer an alternative to the overuse of technology, and to provide a setting and a structure for a practice that promotes and protects relationships. From a more principles-based perspective, the justification for hospice tends be offered in terms of autonomy, because it protects a sphere of decisional freedom in terms of patients determining their own care. From a care perspective, on the other hand, hospice functions to provide precisely the sort of focus most people need at the end of life. Rather than only being justified as simply one more option available to a rational chooser, care recognizes that hospice-type care focuses on protecting a space where caring relationships can function, regardless of the level of autonomy available to a patient in the process of dying. The difference between these approaches becomes significant when some of the perennial problems in end of life care are examined.

Surveys in recent years have indicated that although a majority of patients would prefer to die in either a hospice-type institutional setting or in their own homes, many of them are not informed of the options in a sufficiently timely manner to allow for the necessary transfer of care. By the time they realize that they are in the process of dying, they are already so weakened that they are unable to make the transfer to another facility, and they end up spending their final days in an acute care setting, receiving the sort of high-technology care that both decreases quality of life and increases costs (Freund et al., 2012; Huskamp et al., 2009; Thomas et al., 2009). The most significant variable in determining whether or not patients enter hospice is communication with their physician; having a discussion about hospice care significantly increases use of hospice services.

Framing patient care in terms of rights and autonomous choices is one of the underlying factors in this frustrating dynamic. So long as good care is understood as a matter of the proper use of the technological and pharmaceutical and surgical resources available in the health care context, guided by a physician's expert knowledge to ensure that all are used with the greatest expertise possible, and in each case affirmed by a patient exercising informed consent that accords with the expert's opinion, so long as that is the picture of care that structures decisions, hospice will remain just one more option among many in end of life care. Obviously, all relevant options should be discussed with patients, but given the limitations of time and patient attention span, any discussion of options needs to be narrowed to a few top choices; hospice may or may not be among those options. And so long as patients are given a reasonable range of options from which to choose, the physician has done his or her duty.

If, on the other hand, patient care is instead framed in terms of providing care that protects and maintains the relational context that keeps a patient connected in important emotional and social ways to his or her family network, then the emphasis on autonomy and the right to choose, while still vitally important, becomes a means to an end, not an end in itself. Offering only options that do not accommodate relational connections can be seen as the failure of care that it is, not a simple matter of adequately offering a range of choices for treatment modalities. But seeing this requires recognizing that aiming at any of the goals of medicine, whether the goal of health or alleviation of pain or a peaceful death, requires a concomitant understanding of the particular person and his or her social context. Health is not just a matter of what an autonomous individual may choose; it is a complex matter of physical, mental, and spiritual connections maintained and protected. Alleviation of pain cannot be just a matter of providing analgesics; it requires addressing spiritual and psychological distress, especially in the context of an individual facing death. A peaceful death may require some hard conversations and emotional distress before real peace can be found.

Care theory thus offers a context for careful thought about how to aim for the various goals of medicine that is particularly apt for end of life care because it situates patients (and caregivers) in the midst of a vital relational network, one that is particular to the patient and her or his circumstances, and one that cannot be simply defined in terms of autonomous choices among an array of options. What the options are needs to be considered, since one can have an array of options, none of which really address the need to maintain connections during the end of one's life.

One of the interesting features of hospice, in fact, is that it addresses so many of the issues we have examined during the course of this book. Rather than working with the assumption that ever more complicated and expensive treatment protocols will improve end of life care, hospice makes the use of technology submit to the achievement of other goals. New medical capacities and procedures are not dismissed. The palliative care incorporated into hospice treatment generally uses the most current pain control techniques possible, and does not require patients to forego other sorts of technology. But the technology is not an end in itself. It serves the needs of those who are in the process of dying, which changes the way it is used.

In a similar manner, the notion of expertise in hospice care also changes. Hospice makes extensive use of lay volunteers, nurses, therapists, and family members as 'expert caregivers' working alongside the more traditional physician authority figures. Again, it is not that physicians have no role to play—they are vital members of the hospice team. But physicians are treated as one expert among many, skilled in the techniques and knowledge of pain control, for example, but not so expert in working with family dynamics or teaching family members how to provide care. Hospice requires a team approach to be successful, and the non-technical members of the team (therapists, social workers, chaplains) are often among the most important members.

Due to its alternative focus, hospice also is far less expensive to operate than traditional 'do everything' end of life care. A dying patient can receive fantastic amounts of intervention, and the cost of end of life care reflects the many things that medicine can offer. Unfortunately, the extensive use of every intervention possible generally does very little to make a patient's last days comfortable or supportive. The more surgeries and complicated machinery caregivers employ, the less comfort and the more isolation patients experience. Spending more money does not necessarily correlate with better care in this case; paying attention to the actual needs of the whole person produce far better care, and far better experiences for the whole family.

From the perspective of an ethics of care, there is a lesson here for the rest of medical practice. The lesson is neither that technology should be done away with, nor that spending money on health care is a bad idea, obviously, but rather that the use of both technology and money needs to be focused on the actual needs of particular, interdependent people (Eckenwiler, 2012). There are appropriate times to spend money and use complex, technologically advanced treatments, but the mere fact that the technology is there does not always justify its use. A focus on the actual needs of particular people, however, requires a very different set of skills than are often thought of as central to medical practice.

End of Life Care and Caring Professionals

The last issue I want to discuss in this chapter is the way that end of life care allows us to see how the social structures of medicine may develop caregivers who find it difficult to provide good care. At the beginning of this book, in discussing an ethics of care, I noted the central importance care ethics places on who one is, rather than what one knows. In discussions about why patients are not referred to hospice at an early enough stage to really benefit from its resources, one regularly finds that the physicians in charge of the patient's care chose not to bring up the topic, often because they equate it with telling a patient to give up. In some cases, physicians thought they had covered the possibility of hospice as one among several treatment options, but patients missed or failed to hear that part of the discussion. In some cases, the physicians in charge of patient care did not realize that it was time for a discussion of hospice for a variety of reasons, and so failed to bring it up.

It should not be surprising that we find this situation. As already noted, the shape that the structures of medicine create, especially in the acute care setting, focus the attention of caregivers on everything but the sort of supportive care that hospice provides. Technological brilliance focuses caregivers' attention on all the wonderful things that can be done for patients; the power structures of medicine make those with the most technical skills and advanced knowledge of available treatments the authorities in the health care setting; the economic structures of medicine are set up reward treatment protocols, not (say) sitting by a bedside listening to a patient; and even the very structure of knowledge is geared toward positive outcomes, usually measured by improved physical condition or some other measurable variable.

Those who work in this context are acutely conscious of the ways that all these factors can enhance care, which makes it difficult to remember that they can also undermine the capacity to provide care. The social structures within which we work shape our experiences, focus our attention, and shape us into certain types of people.

Consider how the hierarchy of medical structures shapes people's perception of their own and others' authority. Medical authority is linked very closely to abstract knowledge. The more one knows, abstractly, about complex and difficult medical conditions, the higher one's status and authority. In contrast, the more one's knowledge is of the practical, hands-on variety, the lower one's status (Anspach, 1993). Physicians thus have more status than nurses, who in turn are ranked above aides and orderlies. Among physicians, those with the greatest degree of specialization have a higher ranking than those with generalist degrees. With the advent of EBP as the paradigm for knowledge and expertise, the knowledge in question has become even more a matter of abstract generalizations and statistical probabilities than it was with a clinical judgment model, which at the very least still required a practitioner to have developed extensive clinical experience with actual patients.

There are good reasons for this basic structure—noting it is not to automatically condemn it. Personally, I am generally happy to be treated by practitioners with extensive knowledge of my condition, and with the research skills to figure out what they don't yet know. The knowledge is not problematic in and of itself, but it becomes problematic because of the way it tends to edge out other sources of knowledge, and to demote the ways of gaining understanding that are often central to practices of care.

Caring for the physical and psycho-social needs of patients can generate the capacity to see and recognize aspects of patient care that are not so easily visible from the heights of abstract statistical studies. When one spends time talking with a white Midwestern family struggling to make decisions about their 8-year-old with an inoperable tumor, one realizes the importance of spending time waiting for people to think through what they need to know. Information is, of course, important, but they need much more than information. They also need to be told that if they want to call in a pastor or church members to sit with them, that would be fine. Going it alone is a really bad idea at a time like this. They may need assurance that their child's condition is not God's punishment, and that other children don't need to be kept away because the condition isn't contagious. Most of all, they will probably need someone to sit down with them and talk about what to expect in the days and months ahead, and who to call when decisions feel too weighty.

Discussions of this sort are not always well performed by highly educated oncology specialists. Chaplains, social workers, nurses, and psychologists tend to be better able to work through these sorts of issues in ways that provide supportive care in a gentle and effective manner. The knowledge of how to carry out a conversation of this sort is clearly as central to providing good care as is the specialized medical knowledge of the oncologist, but it tends to be treated as secondary and less important because of the way authority and knowledge are structured in a health care setting. Because of the way that these social structures shape the medical context, in fact, it is frequently the case that personal knowledge is not seen as knowledge at all, even by those most skilled at helping patients deal with these difficult issues. Instead it is often treated as 'instinct' or as 'being a nice person' rather than recognized for what it is.

Authority and knowledge are not the only social structures that shape medical practice, of course. But the other structures discussed in this book tend to shape medical care in much the same ways as knowledge and power. Economic forces track epistemic prestige quite closely. The more specialized one's knowledge is generally considered to be, the more highly one is rewarded economically. Conversely, the more time one spends actually talking to or touching patients, the less one is likely to be paid, and the less one's work with patients is seen as central to good medical care. Ironically, in fact, it is generally far easier to get insurance companies to pay for specialists than for basic care and ongoing therapy, in spite of that fact that the latter are far cheaper than the former.

I am not the first to note that ways that the structures of medicine can shape the way that care is given in problematic ways, and a number of solutions have been proposed and attempted. The loss of empathy in medical students has been documented and analyzed extensively (Hojat et al., 2009) In response, medical schools have implemented a number of programs designed to improve physician empathy and bedside manners. Some medical schools require physicians in training to experience for themselves some aspect of what their patients experience. One innovative program used temporary tattoos to teach medical students what living with psoriasis was like, for example (Latham et al., 2012). Other schools require journaling throughout the first year of medical school, ethics classes, or learning basic features of empathy (Elmore, 2011). It is hard to know how effective programs of this sort are, though there is some evidence that experiential programs may be somewhat more likely to produce physicians able to interact with patients in ways that convey understanding and care than programs that rely on intellectual understanding of the nature of empathy. In any case, however, the need for such programs indicates a recognition that medical education is structured in ways that reduce empathy, and that this is a problem.

What may be needed, however, is a broader recognition of the ways that the various structures of medicine interact to encourage medical professionals to become cold, distant, or uncaring people. To some degree, every medical professional needs to learn emotional distancing. Over-involvement in the emotional lives of patients is a major factor in burnout, and professionals need to learn how to care for patients without taking on all their emotional baggage. But the social structures of medicine that we have been examining can exert a pressure that takes a reasonable level of emotional distance and pushes it further into overt coldness or inability to respond in caring ways, or that makes caregivers pay a heavy emotional toll if they do continue to care for their patients.

EBP, for example, can improve interactions between caregivers and patients to the degree that it levels hierarchies of knowledge, allowing both caregivers and patients to see and respect each other's capacity to understand a particular condition or develop specialized knowledge of a particular disease. One often sees this sort of respect between caregivers and patients or families who have formed support groups, keep up with the latest research, and know as much as they can about their condition. At the same time, because knowledge is framed in terms of fairly specialized understanding of statistical data, other ways of knowing that may involve more personal or empathetic understanding can disappear. This, in fact, seems to be part of the dynamic in medical school, where the emphasis on knowing every detail of any given condition makes it more difficult for residents to respond to patients at an emotional level. Their training focuses so heavily on facts, statistics, and treatment possibilities that any other aspect of diagnosis or disease disappears from consciousness.

In my own experience on ethics committees, I have found over the years that one of the comments I make, over and over again, week after week, is that the care team needs to get the hospital chaplains or social workers involved in whatever case we are discussing. Caregivers and family find themselves at loggerheads, and no one has thought to call in the chaplains to pray with the patient, to ask about their spiritual situation, to talk about why they insist that life support be kept on because God might still perform a miracle; or the patient is difficult and uncooperative, but no one has thought to bring in the social worker to address cultural factors that make this patient extremely uncomfortable with any men in the room. These aren't cases wherein the problem is a lack of medical knowledge. The professionals are well-informed, keep up on changes in their field, and know where to find all the latest research on particular conditions, but that picture of what it means to be knowledgeable seems to sometimes put blinders on when it comes to issues that are outside the domain of meta-studies of treatment protocols.

Just as the way knowledge is framed can make it hard to see and empathize with other concerns of the patient, the way that economic structures in health care function to focus attention and limit access can also affect caregivers as people. In Chapter 3, I noted the way that economic models of efficiency squeeze nurses away from attending to the holistic needs of their patients. I also noted the way that funding patterns (reimbursement directed toward technology, rather than toward human contact) forces medical care into a certain shape. I will not reiterate those discussions here, though they are clearly relevant. Instead, I want to note another significant way that economic structures affect the character of medical professionals. The first is the way that lack of access to payment affects the caregiver/patient relationship.

When certain patients need regular medical treatment, and are simply unable to pay for it, their arrival (at an emergency room, at a med center, or the like) represents not only a claim on the time and attention of the caregivers. It also represents yet another occasion for busy professionals to set aside the overwhelming tasks they already need to take care of in order to figure out how to find funding to cover this individual's care. It is to their credit that most health care professionals do not try to simply avoid providing care altogether (though occasional anecdotes of this do occur), but rather make the effort to find some way of providing treatment, even in the absence of insurance, Medicaid, or any other payment source.

But the relationship between caregivers and these patients can be particularly frustrating and fraught. It is hard to see a person who consistently asks for (or demands) treatment but has no means for paying for it as anything other than a sponger or a parasite. If the patient has a chronic problem (as is often the case), their regular presentation at an emergency room is likely to gain them the title of a frequent flier. Needing to provide regular care to individuals who seem parasitical, constantly in need, and unable to take minimal steps to provide for their own care leaves many caregivers jaded and frustrated, unwilling or unable to meet this (and perhaps the next patient) with respect or trust. While some of this frustration is simply the expected outcome of dealing with a population that can be difficult (people living in very marginal circumstances, often struggling with untreated psychological conditions, are difficult to deal with at the best of times), the added factor of economic pressure makes it that much more difficult for health care workers to maintain an attitude of care and respect.

Economics is a measure of worth in a capitalist culture such as that of the US, and the needy are increasingly vilified in the political rhetoric of the day. This basic measure of the worth of a person cannot but inform the perspective health care professionals take toward their various patients. If an economic system has large gaps in coverage, there will almost of necessity be certain demographics who cannot pay for the care they need, and must enter the system as supplicants of some sort. And setting up the relationship in that particular configuration affects how caregivers see themselves, as well as their patients, splitting the patient population into the deserving and the undeserving, the worthy and the spongers.

This problem may be resolved to some degree as the US moves toward a broader system of coverage with the Affordable Care Act. But any economic structure affects those functioning within it, and while this problem may lessen with a broader funding base, others may begin to surface. For example, in single-payer systems with a limit on the funds available to a regional health care system, quiet, unmentioned rationing often becomes the norm. No specific policies are set, but caregivers simply don't offer certain types of treatment to certain types of patients (joint replacement to the elderly, for example). In such a system, caregivers become accustomed to making decisions about patients that can be paternalistic, or that rely on judgments about the patient's life and interests that can simply be wrong. But the patient doesn't have the opportunity to challenge misperceptions because she or he probably doesn't even know the decision has been made.

Again, economic structures affect relationships, and they affect the character of those who work within the system. No economic system can be free of these effects. The question that faces us is one of recognizing how economics shapes relationships, and of providing structures that counter problematic tendencies. When we think of end of life care, and the economic forces at work in that context, it becomes particularly important to be aware of the ways that economic structures can affect relationships between caregiver and patient, and in so doing, have effects on the character of the caregivers as well.

Two areas of economic activity offer examples of this dynamic. This chapter has been largely positive about the role that hospice can play in changing end of life care. But there can be a more troubling side to the hospice movement. One of the reasons frequently offered for moving to a hospice model for end of life is the potential for keeping the cost of medical treatment at the end of life to a more reasonable level. End of life care accounts for a full quarter of all Medicare expenditures, for example, and it is frequently assumed (though sometimes challenged [Emanuel and Emanuel, 1994]) that providing better access to hospice and palliative care would decrease this percentage, though studies have not found this to be true to date (Riley and Lubitz, 2010). For our purposes, the actual level of savings (or lack thereof) from hospice care is not the central issue, however. What I want to focus on is the fact of choosing to fund hospice because it represents the possibility of saving money.

Clearly, there is nothing wrong with trying to rein in health care costs, and in the case of a practice such as hospice that generates far higher levels of patient satisfaction than, say, dying in the intensive care unit, the combination of cost savings and improved quality of care are a very positive combination. But in the US, many decisions about what services will (or won't) be covered are made by third-party payers, insurance companies which are distanced from both patients and caregivers. As pressure to rein in health care costs mounts, and as decisions about end of life care are increasingly made on the basis of economic efficiency, then, we might expect an increase in the sense among caregivers that patients have a duty to move to hospice at a certain point, that their 'irrational' demands for continued intensive care are illegitimate and selfish.

I should be clear that this is not the current situation, and hospice is, all things considered, a far better way to manage end of life care than the current alternatives. I raise the issue of how end of life care is understood, however, because it has the potential for this sort of a shift in the dynamics of the caregiver/patient relationship, and we need to be aware of that possibility to ensure that it does not become the central framing paradigm for responding to dying patients.

Clearly, the social structures that shape medical practice affect who caregivers are and who they become. From the perspective of an ethics of care, this matters. Medical practice is not just a matter of isolated events and interactions between individuals. It is a complex set of structures that interact in complicated and often unexpected ways to shape the care given to patients, the interactions among professionals, and the relationships that provide the context for care.

Conclusions

My friend's baby continues to survive and grow, with occasional crises of the sort that are relatively standard for such a premature baby. It looks as though the choices she and her husband have been making will be categorized as neonatal care rather than end of life decisions, and we are all hopeful that this will be the case. But her situation reminds us that we simply don't always know which decisions will (eventually) be categorized as end of life decisions, for the simple reason that all end of life care begins as relatively routine care for what appear to be treatable conditions. It becomes end of life care when the conditions turn out to not be treatable, or complications set in, or some other difficulty appears, and the situation shifts from one likely scenario to another. Just where that tipping point occurs is very difficult to identify when one is in the midst of making decisions—it only becomes clear in retrospect after one know what the outcome turned out to be.

Because of that, and while I am a huge proponent of hospice, I am also sympathetic to the many caregivers who are criticized for not encouraging hospice use earlier, or to the many patients who are resistant to the notion of hospice when it is raised. The shift from thinking of medical care as aiming at restoring function or curing a condition to aiming at palliative care and comfort in dying is not one that happens easily or quickly. To the extent that hospice is presented as a modality of treatment that truly serves the patient's best interests in many cases, that represents good care in both the medical and the ethical sense, however, I believe it is easier to broach the possibility of hospice as for the good of the patient.

If, however, hospice becomes a protocol designed mostly to diminish end of life costs, and this is understood as its primary benefit, then my sense is that resistance to hospice will not only begin to grow, but that it should be resisted. The goal of care needs to be the good of the patient, not first and foremost the financial best interests of an insurance company, or control of medical resources by other professionals. In this area, as in so much of medical practice, we need to learn to accept the limits of our knowledge and our capacities, recognizing that any and all care will always be given under conditions of uncertainty and finitude. As long as there is this level of uncertainty about whether or not one even is at the end of life, pronouncements about how treatment ought to be given in the context need to be tempered with a recognition that people frequently don't know that their situation is an end of life case.

This uncertainty and finitude also reminds us of the vital importance of creating structures of care sufficiently flexible to meet patient needs in the middle of confusion and lack of clarity. Structures that provide for ample feedback and discussion between caregivers and patients, that protect patients from the demands of rigid protocol, and that honor the various types of knowledge brought to the situation by all those involved are structures that allow for far better care to be given. Conversely, sharply limited conceptions of what real knowledge is, rigidly enforced hierarchical structures, and inflexible and bureaucratic economic systems work against the provision of good care. These latter also generate enormous pressure on caregivers to become something other than the caring, responsive selves that they usually want to be. Care becomes so difficult in the context of badly formed structures that caregivers are almost forced to stop caring in order to stay sane.

The social structures of contemporary medicine are not, of course, so badly put together that care is no longer possible. Aspects of the current social structures work tremendously well for providing care, generally very good care. But there are also aspects of the way we organize medicine that can make caregiving more difficult or needlessly complicated, and it is worth identifying those aspects so that their effects can be controlled or mitigated.

Note

1 Truth-telling in medicine is a central component in many standard bioethics texts. (See, for example, Veatch, 2002; Munson, 2004; Jonsen et al., 1982.) For an overview of the historical controversies over truth-telling, see Sokol (2006). Cultural differences in expectations about truth-telling continue to generate discussion and debate, particularly about how to respond to patients from cultures that do not expect truth-telling in a context shaped by the legalities of informed consent and advanced planning procedures for end-of life care. See, for example, Crow et al. (2000) and Candib (2002).

Bibliography

Abellanoza, Adrian, Nicolette Provenzano-Hass, and Robert Gatchel. (2018). "Burnout in ER nurses: Review of the literature and interview themes" *Journal of Applied Biobehavior Research* 23(1). https://doi.org/10.1111/jabr.12117

Aberg, Judith, Joel Blankson, Jeanne Marrazzo, and Adaora Adimora. (2017). "Diversity in the US infectious diseases workforce: Challenges for women and underrepresented minorities" *The Journal of Infectious Diseases* 216(Suppl 5): S606–S610.

Adriaenssens, Jef, Véronique De Gucht, and Stan Maes. (2015). "Determinants and prevalence of burnout in emergency nurses: A systematic review of 25 years of research" *Nursing Studies* 52(2): 649–661.

Aiken, Linda, Sean Clarke, Douglas Sloane, Julie Sochalski, Reinhard Busse, Heather Clarke, Phyllis Giovannetti, Jennifer Hunt, Anne Marie Rafferty, and Judith Shamian. (2001). "Nurses' reports on hospital care in five countries" *Health Affairs* 20(3): 43–53.

Aiken, Linda, Sean Clarke, Douglas Sloane, Julie Sochalski, and Jeffrey Silber. (2002). "Hospital nurse staffing and patient mortality, nurse burnout, and job dissatisfaction" *JAMA* 288 (16): 1987–1993.

Allen, Jane. (2011). "Two dead since Arizona Medicaid program slashed transplant coverage" *ABC News Medical Unit* January 6.

American College of Physicians. (2008). "Achieving a high performance health care system with universal access: What the US can learn from other countries" *Annals of Internal Medicine* 148(1): 55–75.

Anand, Sudhir, and Kara Hanson. (2004). "Disability-adjusted life years: A critical review" in *Public Health, Ethics, and Equity*, Sudhir Anand, Fabienne Peter, and Amartya Sen, eds. Oxford: Oxford University Press, pp. 183–199.

Angell, Marcia. (2008). "Privatizing health care is not the answer: Lessons from the United States" *CMAJ* 179(9): 916–919.

Anspach, Renée. (1993). *Deciding Who Lives: Fateful Choices in the Intensive-Care Nursery*. Berkeley: University of California Press.

Asgeirsdóttir, T.L., G. Asmundsdóttir, M. Heimisdóttir, E. Jónsson, and R. Pálsson. (2009). "Cost effectiveness analysis for end-stage renal disease" (article in Icelandic) *Laeknabladid* 95(11): 747–753.

Baier, Annette. (1994). *Moral Prejudices: Essays on Ethics*. Cambridge, MA: Harvard University Press.

Barnes, William, Myles Gartland, and Martin Stack. (2004). "Old habits die hard: Path dependency and behavioral lock-in" *Journal of Economic Issues* 38(2): 371–377.

Baron, Charles. (1983). "Licensure of health care professionals: The consumer's case for abolition" *American Journal of Law and Medicine* 335–356.

Beauvoir, Simone de. (1952). *The Second Sex.* H.M. Parshley, trans. New York: Alfred A. Knopf.

Becker, Marshall. (1985). "Patient adherence to prescribed therapies" *Medical Care* 23(5): 539–555.

Benhabib, Seyla. (1992). *Situating the Self: Gender, Community, and Postmodernism in Contemporary Ethics.* New York: Routledge.

Benner, Patricia, Patricia Hooper Kyriakidis, and Daphne Stannard. (2011). *Clinical Wisdom and Interventions in Acute and Critical Care: A Thinking-in-Action Approach,* 2nd ed. New York: Springer Publishing Company.

Bentley, T. Scott, and Steven Phillips. (2017). "2017 U.S. organ and tissue transplant cost estimates and discussion" *Milliman Research Report.* http://us.milliman.com/uploadedFiles/insight/2017/2017-Transplant-Report.pdf

Berk, Marc, and Alan Monheit. (2001). "The concentration of health care expenditures, revisited" *Health Affairs* 20(2): 9–18. http://content.healthaffairs.org/content/20/2/9.short

Betsch, Cornelia, Corina Ulshöfer, Frank Renkewitz, and Tilmann Betsch. (2011). "The influence of narrative v. statistical information on perceiving vaccination risks" *Medical Decision Making* 31(5): 742–753.

Bialik, Carl. (2010). "Health studies cited for transplant cuts put under the knife" *Wall Street Journal* December 18.

Bishop, Anne, and John Scudder. (1991). *Nursing: The Practice of Caring.* New York: National League for Nursing Press.

Blagg, Christopher. (2007). "The early history of dialysis for chronic renal failure in the United States: A view from Seattle" *American Journal of Kidney Diseases* 49(3): 482–496.

Blazheski, Filip, and Nathaniel Karp. (2018). "Got symptoms? High U.S. healthcare spending and its long-term impact on economic growth" *U.S. Economic Watch* March 29 (BBVA Research). www.bbvaresearch.com/wp-content/uploads/2018/03/180329_US_HealhcareCosts.pdf

Blendon, Robert J., Minah Kim, and John M. Benson. (2001). "The public versus the world health organization on health system performance" *Health Affairs* 20(3): 10–20.

Boamah, Sheila, Emily Read, and Health Laschinger. (2017). "Factors influencing new graduate nurse burn-out development, job satisfaction and patient care quality: A time-lagged study" *Journal of American Nursing* 73(5): 1182–1195.

Booth, P.M., and G.M. Dickinson. (1998). "Public or private? Insurance and Pensions" in *Health Care, Ethics, and Insurance,* Tom Sorrell, ed. New York: Routledge, pp. 181–215.

Boyd, Cynthia, Jonathan Darer, Chad Boult, Minda Fried, Lisa Boult, and Albert Wu. (2005). "Clinical practice guidelines and quality of care for older patients with multiple co-morbid diseases: Implications for pay for performance" *JAMA* 294(6): 716–724.

Boykin, Anne, and Savina Schoenhofer. (1993). *Nursing as Caring: A Model for Transforming Practice*. New York: National League for Nursing Press.

Brabeck, Mary. (1993). "Moral judgment: Theory and research on differences between males and females" in *An Ethics of Care: Feminist and Interdisciplinary Perspectives*. Mary Jeanne Larrabee, ed. New York: Routledge.

Breyer, Friedrich, and Stefan Felder. (2006). "Life expectancy and health care expenditures: A new calculation for Germany using the costs of dying" *Health Policy* 75(2): 178–186. www.sciencedirect.com/science/article/pii/S0168851005000680

Bright, Cedric, Mia Price, Randall Morgan, and Rahn Bailey. (2018). "The report of the W. Montague Cobb/NMA health institute consensus panel on the plight of underrepresented minorities in medical education" *Journal of the National Medical Association* Available online June 5, 2018, in press. https://doi.org/10.1016/j.jnma.2018.03.012

Brock, Dan. (2004). "Ethics issues in the use of cost effectiveness analysis for the prioritization of health care resources" in *Public Health, Ethics, and Equity*, Sudhir Anand, Fabienne Peter, and Amartya Sen, eds. Oxford: Oxford University Press, pp. 201–223.

Brody, David. (1980). "The patient's role in clinical decision-making" *Annals of Internal Medicine* 93(5): 718–722.

Brody, Howard. (1992). *The Healer's Power*. New Haven: Yale University Press.

Brody, Howard. (2009). *The Future of Bioethics*. Oxford: Oxford University Press.

Brown, Melissa, Gary Brown, and Sanjay Sharma. 2005. *Evidence-Based to Value Based Medicine*. Chicago: AMA Press.

Bubeck, Diemut. (1995). *Care, Gender, Justice*. New York: Clarendon Press.

Buetow, S., and T. Kenealy. (2000). "Evidence-based medicine: The need for a new definition" *Journal of Evaluation and Clinical Practice* 6(2): 85–92.

Callahan, Daniel. (1992). "Reforming the health care system for children and the elderly to balance cure and care" *Academic Medicine* 67(4): 219–221.

Callahan, Daniel. (2009). *Taming the Beloved Beast: How Medical Technology Costs Are Destroying Our Health Care System*. Princeton: Princeton University Press.

Candib, Lucy. (2002). "Truth telling and advance planning at the end of life: Problems with autonomy in a multicultural world" *Families, Systems, & Health* 20(3): 213–228.

Card, Claudia. (1995). "Gender and moral luck" in *Justice and Care: Essential Readings in Feminist Ethics*. Virginia Held, ed. Boulder, CO: Westview Press.

Cassell, Eric. (1998). "The nature of suffering and the goals of medicine" *Loss, Grief and Care* 8(1–2): 129–142.

CDC. (2016). "2016 Fertility clinic success rates report" https://www.cdc.gov/art/artdata/index.html

Chambliss, Daniel. (1996). *Beyond Caring: Hospitals, Nurses, and the Social Organization of Ethics*. Chicago: University of Chicago Press.

Chin, Weishan, Yue-Liang Leon Guo, Yu-Ju Hung, Yuh-Tzu Hseih, Li-Jie Wang, and Judith Shu-Chu Shiao. (2017). "Workplace justice and intention to leave the nursing profession" *Nursing Ethics* 1–13.

Code, Lorraine. (1991). *What Can She Know? Feminist Theory and the Construction of Knowledge*. Ithaca: Cornell University Press.

Code, Lorraine. (2015). "Care, concern, and advocacy: Is there a place for epistemic responsibility?" *Feminist Philosophy Quarterly* 1(1): 1–20.

Coleman, Carl. (2002). "Conceiving harm: Disability discrimination in assisted reproductive technologies" *UCLA Law Review* 50: 101–156.

Collins, Patricia Hill. (2000). *Black Feminist Thought: Knowledge, Consciousness, and the Politics of Empowerment*, 2nd ed. New York: Routledge.

Corea, Gena, Renate Duelli Klein, Jalna Hammer, Helen B. Holmes, Betty Hoskins, Madhu Kishwar, Janice Raymond, Robyn Rowland, and Roberta Steinbacher. (1987). *Man-Made Women: How New Reproductive Technologies Affect Women.* Indianapolis: Indiana University Press.

Coverdill, James, Alfredo Carbonello, Jonathan Fryer, George Fuhrman, Kristi Harold, Jonathan Hiatt, Benjamin Jarman, Richard Moore, Don Nakayama, Timothy Nelson, Marc Schlatter, Richard Sidwell, John Tarpley, Paula Termuhlen, Christopher Wohltman, and John Mellinger. (2010). "A new professionalism? Surgical residents, duty hours restrictions, and shift transitions" *Academic Medicine* 85(10): S72–S75.

Cox, A. C., L. J. Fallowfield, and V. A. Jenkins. (2006). "Communication and informed consent in phase 1 trials: A review of the literature" *Support Care Cancer* 14: 303–309.

Coyne, Cathy, Ronghui Xu, Peter Raich, Kathy Plomer, Mark Dignan, Lari Wenzel, Diane Fairclough, Thomas Habermann, Linda Schnell, Susan Quella, and David Cella. (2003). "Randomized, controlled trial of an easy-to-read informed consent statement for clinical trial participation: A study of the Eastern Cooperative Oncology Group" *Journal of Clinical Oncology* (March 1) 21(5): 836–842.

Crow, Karine, Lou Mattheson, and Alicia Steed. (2000). "Informed consent and truth-telling: Cultural directions for health care providers" *The Journal of Nursing Administration* 30(3): 148–152.

Cutler, David M., and Mark McClellan. (2001). "Is technological change in medicine worth it?" *Health Affairs* 20(5): 11–29.

Daniels, Norman. (1985). *Just Health Care.* Cambridge: Cambridge University Press.

Dellasega, Cheryl. (2009). "Bullying among nurses" *American Journal of Nursing* 109(1): 52–58. doi:10.1097/01.NAJ.0000344039.11651.08

De Valk, Chris, Jozien Bensing, R. Bruynooghe, and V. Batenburg. (2001). "Cure oriented versus care oriented attitudes in medicine" *Patient Education and Counseling* 45(2): 119–126.

DeVries, Raymond, Lisa Kane Lowe, and Elizabeth (Libby) Bogdan-Lovis. (2009). "Choosing surgical birth: Desires and the nature of bioethical advice" in *Naturalized Bioethics: Toward Responsible Knowing and Practice.* Cambridge: Cambridge University Press, pp. 42–64.

Dewar, Diane. (2010). *Essentials of Health Economics.* Sudbury, MA: Jones & Bartlett.

Dickenson, Donna. (2001). "Property and women's alienation from their own reproductive labour" *Bioethics* 15(3): 205–217.

Doucet, Andrea. (2017). "The ethics of care and the radical potential of fathers 'Home Alone on Leave': Care as practice, relational ontology, and social justice" in *Comparative Perspectives on Work-Life Balance and Gender Equality*, M. O'Brien and K. Wall, eds. New York: Springer International, pp. 11–28.

Eckenwiler, Lisa A. (2012). *Long-Term Care, Globalization, and Justice.* Baltimore: The Johns Hopkins University Press.

Elmore, Shekinah. (2011). "The good doctor" *The Journal of the American Medical Association* (October 12) 306(14): 1525–1526.

Elshtain, Jean Bethke. (1981). *Public Man, Private Woman: Women in Social and Political Thought*, 2nd ed. Princeton: Princeton University Press.

Emanuel, Ezekiel, and Linda Emanuel. (1994). "The economics of dying—The illusion of cost savings at the end of life" *New England Journal of Medicine* (February 24) 330: 540–544.

Engster, Daniel. (2007). *The Heart of Justice: Care Ethics and Political Theory.* Oxford: Oxford University Press.

Engster, Daniel, and Maurice Hamington, eds. (2015). *Care Ethics and Political Theory.* Oxford: Oxford University Press.

Esserman, Laura, and Margaret O'Kane. (2014). "Moving beyond the breast screening debate" *Journal of Women's Health* 23(8): 629–630.

Files, Julia, Anita Mayer, Marcia Ko, Patricia Friedrich, Marjorie Jenkins, Michael Bryan, Suneela Vegunta, Christopher Wittich, Melissa Lyle, Ryan Melikian, Trevor Duston, Yu-Hui Chang, and Sharonne Hayes. (2017). "Speaker introductions at internal medicine grand rounds: Forms of address reveal gender bias" *Journal of Women's Health* 26(5): 413–419.

Flathman, Richard. (1982). "Power, authority, and rights in the practice of medicine" *Philosophy and Medicine* 12: 105–125.

Fleck, Leonard. (2009). *Just Caring: Health Care Rationing and Democratic Deliberation.* Oxford: Oxford University Press.

Flocke, Susan, William Miller and Benjamin Crabtree. (2002). "Relationships between physician practice style, patient satisfaction, and attributes of primary care" *Journal of Family Practice* 51(10): 835.

Flood, Colleen, Kent Roach, and Lorne Sossin, eds. (2005). *Access to Care, Access to Justice: The Legal Debate Over Private Health Insurance in Canada.* Toronto: University of Toronto Press.

Flynn, Linda, and Pamela Ironside. (2018). "Burnout and its contributing factors among midlevel academic nurse leaders" *Journal of Nursing Education* 57(1): 28–34.

Folbre, Nancy. (2013). "Reforming care" *Politics and Society* 12: 197–216.

Freund, Katherine, Michelle Weckmann, David Casarett, Kristi Swanson, Mary Brooks, and Ann Broderick. (2012). "Hospice eligibility in patients who dies in a tertiary care unit" *Journal of Hospital Medicine* 7(3): 218–223.

Friedman, Marilyn. (1993). "Beyond caring: The de-moralization of gender" in *An Ethic of Care: Feminist and Interdisciplinary Perspectives*, Mary Jeanne Larrabee, ed. New York: Routledge.

Friedman, Milton. (1962). *Capitalism and Freedom.* Chicago: University of Chicago Press.

Gabbay, John, and Andrée le May. (2011). *Practice-Based Evidence for Healthcare: Clinical Mindlines.* New York: Routledge.

Galbraith, Alison, Stephen Soumerai, Dennis Ross-Degnan, Meredith Rosenthal, Charlene Gay, and Tracy Lieu. (2012). "Delayed and foregone care for families with chronic conditions in high-deductible health plans" *Journal of General Internal Medicine* 27(9): 1105-1111. `doi:10.1007/s11606-011-1970-8

Gardner, Glenn, Christine Collins, Sonya Osborne, Amanda Henderson, and Misha Eastwood. (2009). "Creating a therapeutic environment: A non-randomised controlled trial of a quiet time intervention for patients in acute care" *International Journal of Nursing Studies* 46(6): 778–786.

Garrosa, Eva, Bernardo Moreno-Jiménez, Alfredo Rodríguez-Muñoz, and Raquel Rodríguez-Carvajal. (2011). "Role stress and personal resources in nursing: A cross-sectional study of burnout and engagement" *International Journal of Nursing Studies* 48(4): 479–489.

Gilligan, Carol. (1982). *In a Different Voice: Psychological Theory and Women's Development*. Cambridge, MA: Harvard University Press.

Gilson, Erinn. (2014). *The Ethics of Vulnerability: A Feminist Analysis of Social Life and Practice*. New York: Routledge.

Giordano, Cristiana. (2018). "Political therapeutics: Dialogues and frictions around care and cure" *Medical Anthropology* 37(1): 32–44.

Glen, Evelyn Nakano. (2010). *Forced to Care: Coercion and Caregiving in America*. Cambridge, MA: Harvard University Press.

Glouberman, Sholom, and Henry Mintzberg. (2001). "Managing the care of health and the cure of disease—part I: Differentiation" *Health Care Management Review* 26(1): 56–69.

Goldberg, Daniel. (2011). "Eschewing definitions of the therapeutic misconception: A family resemblance analysis" *Journal of Medicine and Philosophy* 36(3): 296–320.

Goldstein, Nathan, Lewis Cohen, Robert Arnold, Elizabeth Goy, Stephen Arons, and Linda Gazini. (2012). "Prevalence of formal accusations of murder and euthanasia against physicians" *Journal of Palliative Medicine* (March) 15(3): 334–339.

Gozalo, Pedro, Joan Teno, Susan Mitchell, Jon Skinner, Julie Bynum, Denise Tyler, and Vincent Mor. (2011). 'End of life transitions among nursing home residents with cognitive issues" *New England Journal of Medicine* (September 29) 365: 1212–1221.

Green, Karen. (1995). *The Woman of Reason: Feminism, Humanism, and Political Thought*. New York: Continuum.

Greenhalgh, Trisha. (2010). *How to Read a Paper: The Basics of Evidence-Based Medicine*, 4th ed. New York: BMJ Books.

Greenhalgh, Trisha, Jeremy Howick, and Neal Maskrey. (2014). "Evidence-based medicine: A movement in crisis?" *BMJ* 348: g3725.

Gresenz, Carole, David Studdert, Nancy Campbell, and Deborah Hensler. (2011). "Patients in conflict with managed care: A profile of appeals in two HMOs" *Health Affairs* (March) 30: 3519–3524.

Groenhout, Ruth. (2004). *Connected Lives: Human Nature and an Ethics of Care*. Lanham, MD: Rowman & Littlefield.

Groenhout, Ruth. (2015). "Of medicine and monsters: rationing and an ethics of care" in *Care Ethics and Political Theory*, Daniel Engster and Maurice Hamington, eds. New York: Oxford University Press, pp. 146–164.

Groopman, Jerome. (2007). *How Doctors Think*. New York: Houghton Mifflin.

Gruber, Jonathan, and Maria Owings. (1994). "Physician financial incentives and cesearean section delivery" NBER Working Paper No. 4933. www.nber.org/papers/w4933

Grumbach, Kevin, and Thomas Bodenheimer. (2004). "Can health care teams improve primary care practice?" *JAMA* 291(10): 1246–1251.

Gupta, Jyotsna, and Annemiek Richters. (2008). "Embodied subjects and fragmented objects: Women's bodies, assisted reproduction technologies and the right to self-determination" *Bioethical Inquiry* 5: 239–249.

Haberman, Clyde. 2014. "From private ordeal to national fight: The case of Terri Shiavo" *New York Times* April 20, 2014.

Habka, Dany, David Mann, Ronald Landes, and Alejandro Soto-Gutierrez. (2015). "Future economies of liver transplantations: A 20-year cost modeling forecast and the prospect of bioengineering autologous liver grafts" *PLoS One* 10(7): e0131764.

Haddad, Lisa, and Tammy Toney-Butler. (2018). "Nursing, Shortage" [Updated 2018 May 13] in *StatPearls* [Internet]. Treasure Island, FL: StatPearls Publishing, January. www.ncbi.nlm.nih.gov/books/NBK493175/

Hamington, Maurice. (2004). *Embodied Care; Jane Addams, Maurice Merleau-Ponty, and Feminist Ethics*. Chicago: University of Chicago Press.

Hanoch, Yaniv, and Thomas Rice. (2010). "The economics of choice: Lessons from the U.S. health-care market" *Health Expectations* 14(1): 105–112. doi:10.1111/j.1369-7625.2010.00646.x

Halpern, Jodi. (2001). *From Detached Concern to Empathy: Humanizing Medical Practice*. Oxford: Oxford University Press.

Hankivsky, Olena. (2004). *Social Policy and the Ethic of Care*. Vancouver: UBC Press.

Hanson, Mark, and Daniel Callahan, eds. (1999). *The Goals of Medicine: The Forgotten Issues in Health Care Reform*. Washington, DC: Georgetown University Press.

Hartsock, Nancy. (1999). *The Feminist Standpoint Revisited, and Other Essays*. New York: Basic Books.

Harwood, Karey. (2007). *The Infertility Treadmill: Feminist Ethics, Personal Choice, and the Use of Reproductive Technologies*. Chapel Hill: The University of North Carolina Press.

Havens, Donna, Jody Gittell, and Joseph Vasey. (2018). "Impact of relational coordination on nurse job satisfaction, work engagement, and burnout: Achieving the quadruple aim" *Journal of Nursing Administration* 48(3): 132–140.

Hearn, Julie, and Irene Higginson. (1998). "Do specialist palliative care teams improve outcomes for cancer patients? A systematic literature review" *Palliative Medicine* 12(5): 317–332.

Held, Virginia. (1993). *Feminist Morality: Transforming Culture, Society, and Politics*. Chicago: University of Chicago Press.

Held, Virginia. (2006). *The Ethics of Care: Personal, Political, and Global*. Oxford: Oxford University Press.

Hemenway, Daniel, Alice Killen, Suzanne Cashman, Cindy Parks, and William Bicknell. (1990). "Physicians' responses to financial incentives—evidence from a for-profit ambulatory care center" *New England Journal of Medicine* (April 20) 322: 1059–1063.

Heponiem, Tarja, Marko Elovainio, Anne Kouvonen, Anja Noro, Harriet Finne-Soven, and Timo Sinervo. (2012). "Ownership type and team climate in elderly care facilities: The moderating effect of stress factors" *Journal of Advanced Nursing* 68(3): 647–657. doi:10.1111/j.1365-2648.2011.05777.x

Higgins, Linda. (1999). "Nurses' perceptions of collaborative nurse-physician transfer decision making as a predictor of patient outcomes in a medical intensive care unit" *Journal of American Nursing* 29(6): 1434–1443.

Higgs, Joy, Mark Jones, Stephen Loftus, and Nicole Christensen. (2008). *Clinical Reasoning in the Health Professions*, 3rd ed. New York: Butterworth-Heinemann.

Hillman, Alan, Mark Pauly, and Joseph Kerstein. (1989). "How do financial incentives affect physicians' clinical decisions and the financial performance of health maintenancy organizations?" *New England Journal of Medicine* (July 13) 321: 86–92.

Hillyard, Daniel, and Joh Dombrink. (2001). *Dying Right: The Death With Dignity Movement.* New York: Routledge.

Himmelstein, David, Steffie Woolhandler, Mark Almberg, and Clare Fauke. (2018). "The ongoing U.S. health care crisis" *International Journal of Health Services* 48(2): 209–222.

Hojat, Mohammadreza, Michale Vergare, Kaye Maxwell, George Brainard, Steven Herrine, Gerald Isenberg, Jon Veloski, and Joseph Gonnella. (2009). "The devil is in the third year: A longitudinal study of erosion of empathy in medical school" *Academic Medicine* (September) 84(9): 1182–1191.

Howard, K., G. Salkeld, S. White, S. McDonald, S. Chadban, J. C. Craig, and A. Cass. (2009). "The cost effectiveness of increasing kidney transplantation and home-based dialysis" *Nephrology* 14(1): 123–132.

Howick, Jeremy. (2011). *The Philosophy of Evidence-Based Medicine.* New York: Wiley-Blackwell.

Hurst, Samia, Sara Chandros Hull, Gordon DuVal, and Marion Danis. (2005). "Physicians responses to resource constraints" *Archives of Internal Medicine* (March) 165(6): 639–644.

Huskamp, Haiden, Nancy Keating, Jennifer Malin, Alan Zaslavsky, Jane Weeks, Craig Earle, Joan Teno, Beth Viming, Katherine Kahn, Yulei He, and John Ayalian. (2009). "Discussion with physicians about hospice among patients with metastatic lung cancer" *Archives of Internal Medicine* (May) 169(10): 954–962.

Hynes, Patricia, ed. (1991). *Reconstructing Babylon: Essays on Women and Technology.* Indianapolis: Indiana University Press.

Ihde, Don. (1993). *Philosophy of Technology: An Introduction.* New York: Paragon House.

Jacobs, Lawrence, Theodore Marmore, and Jonathan Oberlander. (1999). "The Oregon health plan and the political paradox of rationing: What advocates and critics have claimed and what oregon di" *Journal of Health Politics, Policy and Law* 24(1): 161–180.

Joffe, Steven, E. Francis Cook, and Paul Weeks. (2001). "Quality of informed consent in cancer clinical trials: A cross-sectional survey" *The Lancet* (November) 358(9295): 1772–1777.

Jonsen, Albert. (2007). "The god squad and the origins of transplantation ethics and policy" *The Journal of Law, Medicine, and Ethics* 35(2): 238–240.

Jonsen, Albert, Mark Siegler, and William Winslade. (1982). *Clinical Ethics: A Practical Approach to Ethical Decisions in Clinical Medicine.* New York: Palgrave Macmillan.

Jönsson, B. (2002). "Revealing the cost of Type II diabetes in Europe" *Diabetologia* 45(7): S2–S12. http://link.springer.com/article/10.1007/s00125-002-0858-x

Kachalia, A., S. R. Kaufman, R. Boothman, S. Anderson, K. Welch, S. Saint, and M. A. Rogers. (2010). "Liability claims and costs before and after implementation of a medical error disclosure program" *Annals of Internal Medicine* 153(4): 213–221.

Kaplan, Lawrence, and Rosemarie Tong. (1994). *Controlling our Reproductive Destiny: A Technological and Philosophical Review*. Cambridge, MA: The MIT Press.

Karthikeyan, Ganesan, and Prem Pais. (2009). "Clinical judgment and evidence-based medicine: Time for reconciliation" *The Indian Journal of Medical Research* 132(5): 623–626.

Kass, Leon. (1997). "The wisdom of repugnance" *New Republic* 216(22): 17–26.

Kirch, Darrell, and Kate Petelle. (2017). "Addressing the physician shortage: The peril of ignoring demography" *JAMA* 317(19): 1947–1948.

Kiser, Grace. (2010). *"The Most Outrageous Examples of Health Insurers Denying Coverage"* Huffpost 04/19/2010.

Kittay, Eva Feder. (1999). *Love's Labor: Essays on Women, Equality, and Dependency*. New York: Routledge.

Kittay, Eva Feder, and Ellen K. Feder, eds. (2002). *The Subject of Care: Feminist Perspectives on Dependency*. Lanham, MD: Rowman & Littlefield.

Kitzhaber, J.A. (1993). "Prioritising health services in an era of limits: The Oregon experience" *BMJ* 307: 373–377.

Koehn, Daryl. (1998). *Rethinking Feminist Ethics: Care, Trust, and Empathy*. New York: Routledge.

Koh, Jiwon, Eurah Goh, Kyung-Sang Yu, Belong Cho, and Jeong Hee Yang. (2012). "Discrepancy between participants' understanding and desire to know in informed consent: Are they informed about what they really want to know?" *Journal of Medical Ethics* 38: 102–106.

Kohn, Tamara, and Rosemary McKechnie. (1999). *Extending the Boundaries of Care: Medical Ethics and Caring Practices*. New York: Oxford University Press.

Krakauer, Eric, Christopher Crenner, and Ken Fox. (2002). "Barriers to optimum end-of-life care for minority patients" *Journal of the American Geriatrics Society* 50(1): 182–190.

Kraus, Stephanie, Mark Linzer, Tosha Wetterneck Linda Baier Manwell, Qian Li, and Pascale Carayon. (2011). "Chaotic work environments: Relationship to nursing burnout and intent to leave" *Midwest Nursing Research Society* (October 17). http://hdl.handle.net/10755/160069

Lambda, Sangeeta, and Tammie E. Quest. (2010). "Hospice care and the emergency department: Ruels, regulations and referrals" *Annals of Emergency Medicine* (March) 57(3): 282–290.

Lasser, Karen E., David Himmelstein, and Steffie Woodlander. (2006). "Access to care, health status, and health disparities in the United States and Canada: Results of a cross-national populations-based survey" *American Journal of Public Health* 96(7): 1300–1307.

Latham, Lesley, Aimee MacDonald, Alexa Kimball, and Richard Langley. (2012). "Teaching empathy to undergraduate medical students using a temporary tattoo simulating psoriasis" *Journal of the American Academy of Dermatology* (July) 67(1): 93–99.

Latour, Bruno. (2004). *Politics of Nature: How to Bring the Sciences into Democracy*, Catherine Porter, trans. Cambridge, MA: Harvard University Press.

Lavi, Shai. (2007). *The Modern Art of Dying: A History of Euthanasia in the United States*. Princeton: Princeton University Press.

Ledger, William and Jonathan Skull. 2009. "Rationing fertility services in the NHS: a provider's perspective" *Human Fertility* 3(3): 155-156.

Le Grand, Jukiab. (2009). "Choice and competition in publicly funded health care" *Health Economics, Policy and Law* 4: 479–488. http://dx.doi.org/10.1017/S1744133109990077

Leland, Hayne. (1979). "Quacks, Lemons, and Licensing" *Journal of Political Economy* 87(6): 1328–1346.

Lerner, Gerda. (1993). *The Creation of a Feminist Consciousness: From the Middle Ages to Eighteen-Seventy*. Oxford: Oxford University Press.

Lewis, Malcolm. (2006). "Nurse bullying: Organizational considerations in maintenance and perpetrations of health care bullying cultures" *Journal of Nursing Management* 14(1): 52–58.

Litaker, David, Lorraine Mion, Loretta Planavsky, Christopher Kippes, Neil Mehta, and Joseph Frolkis. (2003). "Physician-nurse practitioner teams in chronic disease management: The impact on costs, clinical effectiveness, and patients' perception of care" *Journal of Interprofessional Care* 17(3): 223–237.

Lockwood, Michael. (1988). "Quality of life and resource allocation" *Philosophy and Medical Welfare* 23: 33–55.

Lorber, Judith. (1992). "Choice, Gift, or Patriarchal Bargain? Women's Consent to *In Vitro* Fertilization in Male Infertility" in *Feminist Perspectives in Medical Ethics*, Helen Bequaert Holmes and Laura Purdy, eds. Bloomington: Indiana University Press.

Lord, Jonathan, Laurence Shaw, Frank Dobbs and Umesh Acharya. (2009). "A time for change and a time for inequality – Infertility services and the NHS" *Human Fertility* 4(4): 256-260.

Lynn, Joanne, and Nathan Goldstein. (2003). "Advance care planning for fatal chronic illness: Avoiding commonplace errors and unwarranted suffering" *Annals of Internal Medicine* 138(10): 812–818.

MacIntyre, Alasdair. (1984). *After Virtue*, 2nd ed. Notre Dame, IN: University of Notre Dame Press.

Mackenzie, Catriona, Wendy Rogers, and Susan Dodds, eds. (2014). *Vulnerability: New Essays in Ethics and Feminist Philosophy*. Oxford: Oxford University Press.

MacKinnon, Catharine. (1987). *Feminism Unmodified: Discourses on Life and Law*. Cambridge, MA: Harvard University Press.

Mackenzie, Catriona, and Natalie Stoljar. (2000). *Relational Autonomy: Feminist Perspectives on Autonomy, Agency, and the Social Self*. Oxford: Oxford University Press.

Mahowald, Mary Briody. (1994). *Philosophy of Woman: An Anthology of Classic to Current Concepts*, 3rd ed. Indianapolis: Hackett Publishing.

Mahowald, Mary Briody. (2000). *Genes, Women, Equality*. Oxford: Oxford University Press.

Malfertheiner, Peter, Francis Chan, and Kenneth McColl. (2009). "Peptic ulcer disease" *The Lancet* 374(9699): 1449–1461.

Manning, Rita. (1992). *Speaking from the Heart: A Feminist Perspective on Ethics*. Lanham, MD: Rowman & Littlefield.

Marquis, Don. (1999). "How to resolve an ethical dilemma concerning randomized clinical trials" *New England Journal of Medicine* 341: 691–693.

May, Elizabeth Tyler. (1995). *Barren in the Promised Land: Childless Americans and the Pursuit of Happiness*. Cambridge, MA: Harvard University Press.

McAlister, Linda Lopez. (1996). *Hypatia's Daughters: Fifteen Hundred Years of Women Philosophers*. Indianapolis: Indiana University Press.

McCullough, Laurence B. (1999). "Moral authority, power, and trust in clinical ethics" *Journal of Medicine and Philosophy* 24(1): 1–3.

McDonagh, Jonathan, Tricia Elliott, Ruth Engelberg, Patsy Treece, Sarah Shannon, Gordon Rubenfeld, Donald Patrick, and Curtis Randall. (2004). "Family satisfaction with family conferences about end-of-life care in the intensive care unit: Increased proportion of family speech is associated with increased satisfaction" *Critical Care Medicine* 32(7): 1484–1488.

McLeod, Carolyn, and Julie Ponesse. (2008). "Infertility and moral luck: The politics of women blaming themselves for infertility" *International Journal of Feminist Approaches to Bioethics* 1(1): 126–144.

McQuillan, Julia, Rosalie Torres Stone, and Arthur Greil. (2007). "Infertility and life satisfaction among women" *Journal of Family Issues* (July) 28(7): 955–981.

Mechanic, David. (1991). "Sources of countervailing power in medicine" *Journal of Health Politics* 16(3): 485–498.

Meunier-Beillard, Nicolas, Auguste Dargent, Fiona Ecarnot, Jean-Philippe Rigaud, Pascal Andreu, Audrey Large, and Jean-Pierre Quenot. (2017). "Intersecting vulnerabilities in professionals and patients in intensive care" *Annals of Translational Medicine* 5(Suppl 4): S39.

Mitchell, Jean. (2008). "Do financial incentives linked to ownership of specialty hospitals affect physicians' practice patterns?" *Medical Care* 46(7): 732–737.

Mohrman, Margaret. (1995). *Medicine as Ministry: Reflections on Suffering, Ethics, and Hope.* Cleveland, OH: Pilgrim Press.

Monsalve-Reyes, Carolina, Concepcion San Luis-Costas, Jose Gomez-Urquiza, Luis Albendin-Garcia, Raimundo Aguayo, and Guillermo Canadas de la Fuente. (2018). "Burnout syndrome and its prevalence in primary care nursing: A systematic review and meta-analysis" *BMC Family Practice* 19: 59. https://doi.org/10.1186/s12875-018-0748-z

Mooney, Gavin. (2009). *Challenging Health Economics.* Oxford: Oxford University Press.

Moore, Susan, Pareen Shenoy, Laura Fanucchi, John Tumeh, and Christopher Flowers. (2009). "Cost-effectiveness of MRI compared to mammography for breast cancer screening in a high risk population" *BMC Health Services Research* 9: 9.

Munnangi, Swapna, Lynore Dupiton, Anthony Boutin, and George Angus. (2018). "Burnout, perceived stress, and job satisfaction among Trauma nurses at a level I safety-net Trauma center" *Journal of Trauma Nursing* 25(1): 4–13.

Munshi, Sunil, Narayanaswamy Vijayakumar, Nicholas Taub, Harneeta Bhullar, T.C. Nelson Lo, and Graham Warwick. (2001). "Outcome of renal replacement therapy in the very elderly" *Nephrology Dialysis Transplantation* 16(1): 128–133.

Munson, Ronald. (2004). *Intervention and Reflection: Basic Issues in Bioethics,* 9th ed. Boston: Wadsworth.

Mussett, Shannon. (2006). "Conditions of servitude: Woman's peculiar role in the master-slave dialectic in Beauvoir's *The Second Sex*" in *The Philosophy of Simone de Beauvoir: Critical Essays,* Margaret A. Simons, ed. Bloomington: Indiana University Press, pp. 276–293.

Myers, Ella. (2013). *Worldly Ethics: Democratic Politics and Care for the World.* Durham: Duke University Press.

Myers, Sara, Katherine Hill, Kristina Nicholson, Matthew Neal, Megan Hamm, Galen Switzer, Leslie Hausmann, Giselle Hamad, Matthew Rosengart, and Eliza Littleton. (2018). "A qualitative study of gender differences in the experiences of general surgery trainees" *Journal of Surgical Research* 228: 127–134.

Narayan, Uma. (1995). "The 'Gift' of a Child: Commercial Surrogacy, Gift Surrogacy, and Motherhood" in *Expecting Trouble: Surrogacy, Fetal Abuse & New Reproductive Technologies*, Patricia Boling, ed. Boulder, CO: Westview Press.

Naugler W.E., and A. Sonnenberg. (2010). "Survival and cost-effectiveness of competing strategies in the management of small hepatocellular carcinoma" *Liver Transplantation* 16(10): 1186–1194.

Neely, Keith, Robert Norton, and Terri Schmidt. (1999). "State insurance commissioner actions against health maintenance organizations for denial of emergency care" *InformaHealth Care* 3(1): 19–22.

NKUDIC (National Kidney and Urological Disease Information Clearing House). (2011). "Kidney and urological disease statistics for the United States" http://kidney.niddk.nih.gov/kudiseases/pubs/kustats/

Noah, Lars. (2003). "Assisted reproductive technologies and the pitfalls of unregulated biomedical innovation" *Florida Law Review* 55(2): 603–635.

Noddings, Nel. (1984). *Caring: A Feminine Approach to Ethics and Moral Education*. Berkeley: University of California Press.

Noddings, Nel. (1989). *Women and Evil*. Berkeley: University of California Press.

Noddings, Nel. (2002). *Starting at Home: Caring and Social Policy*. Berkeley: University of California Press.

Nussbaum, Martha. (2001). *Upheavals of Thought: The Intelligence of Emotions*. Cambridge: Cambridge University Press.

Nye, Andrea. (1988). *Feminist Theory and the Philosophies of Man*. New York: Routledge.

O'Donovan, Oliver. (1984). *Begotten or Made? Human Procreation and Medical Technique*. Oxford: Oxford University Press.

O'Keefe-McCarthy, Sheila. (2009). "Technologically-mediated nursing care and moral agency" *Nursing Ethics* 16(6): 786–796.

Okin, Susan Moller. (1979). *Women in Western Political Thought*. Princeton: Princeton University Press.

Olshansky, E. F. (1996). "A counseling approach with persons experiencing infertility: Implications for advanced practice nursing" *Advanced Practice Nursing Quarterly* 2(3): 42–47.

O'Neill, Onora. (1984). "Paternalism and partial autonomy" *Journal of Medical Ethics* 10(4): 173–178.

Oudshorn, Nelly. (2004). " 'Astronauts in the Sperm World': The renegotiation of masculine identities in discourses on male contraceptives" *Men and Masculinities* 6(4): 349–367.

Papanicolas, Irene, Liana Woskie, and Ashish Jha. (2018). "Health care spending in the United States and other high-income countries" *JAMA* 319(10): 1024–1039.

Papastavrou, Evridiki, Panayiota Andreou, and Georgios Efstathiou. (2013). "Rationing of nursing care and nurse-patient outcomes: a systematic review of quantitative studies" *International Journal of Health Planning and Management* 28(1): 3-25.

Parker, M. (2005). "False dichotomies: EBM, clinical freedom and the art of medicine" *Journal of Medical Ethics* 31: 23–30.

Patel, Vimpla, José Arocha, and David Kaufman. (1999). "Expertise and tacit knowledge in medicine" in *Tacit Knowledge in Professional Practice: Researcher and Practitioner Perspectives*, Robert Sternberg and Joseph Horvath, eds. London: Psychology Press, pp. 75–99.

Pease, Bob. (2018). "Do men care? from uncaring masculinities to men's caring practices in social work" in *Critical Ethics of Care in Social Work: Transforming the Politics and Practices of Caring*, Bob Pease, Anthea Vreugdenhil and Sonya Stanford, eds. New York: Routledge, pp. 186–196.

Pellegrino, Edmund. (1999). "The commodification of medical and health care: The moral consequences of a paradigm shift from a professional to a market ethic" *The Journal of Medicine and Philosophy* 24(3): 243–266.

Petersen, Tove. (2008). Comprehending Care: Problems and Possibilities in the Ethics of Care. Lanham, MD: Lexington Books.

Playle, John, and Philip Keeley. (1998). "Non-compliance and professional power" *Journal of Advanced Nursing* 27: 304–311.

Politi, Mary, and Richard Street. (2010). "The importance of communication in collaborative decision making: Facilitating shared mind and the management of uncertainty" *Journal of Evaluation in Clinical Practice* 17(4): 579–584.

Pols, Jeannette. (2015). "Towards an empirical ethics of care: Relations with technologies in health care" *Medicine, Health Care and Philosophy* 18(1): 81–90.

Polsby, Daniel D. (1998). "Regulation of foods and drugs and Libertarian ideals: Perspectives of a fellow-traveller" in *Problems of Market Liberalism*, Ellen Frankel Paul, Fred D. Miller, and Jeffrey Paul, eds. Cambridge: Cambridge University Press, pp. 209–242.

Poncet, Marie, Philippe Toullic, Laurent Papzian, Nancy Kentish-Barnes, Jean-Francçois Timsit, Frédéric Pochard, Sylie Chevret, Benoît Schlemmer, and Élie Azoulay. (2007). "Burnout dyndrome in critical care nursing staff" *American Journal of Respiratory and Critical Care Medicine* 175(7): 698–704.

Popper-Giveon, Ariela, and Yael Keshet. (2018). "The secret drama at the patient's bedside—refusal of treatment because of the practitioner's ethnic identity: The medical staff's point of view" *Qualitative Health Research* 28(5): 711–720.

Pruthi, Rishi, Sarah Tonkin-Crine, Melania Calestani, Geraldine Leydon, Caroline Eyles, Gabriel Oniscu, Charles Tomson, Andrew Bradley, John Forsythe, Clare Bradley, John Cairns, Christopher Dudley, Christopher Watson, Heather Draper, Rachel Johnson, Wendy Metcalfe, Damien Fogarty, Rommel Ravanan, and Paul Roderick. (2018). "Variation in practice patterns for listing patients for renal transplantation in the United Kingdom: A national survey" *Transplantation* 102(6): 961–968.

Purdy, Alura. (1996). *Reproducing Persons: Issues in Feminist Bioethics*. Ithaca: Cornell University Press.

Quoidbach, Jordi, Elizabeth Dunn, K.V. Petrides, and Moira Mikolajczak. (2010). "Money giveth, money taketh away: The dual effect of wealth on happiness" *Psychological Science* 21(6): 759–763.

Ramsey, Paul. (1970). *Fabricated Man: The Ethics of Genetic Control*. New Haven: Yale University Press.

Rawls, John. (1999). *A Theory of Justice*, rev. ed. Cambridge: Belknap Press.

Reinhardt, Uwe. (2017). "Where does the health insurance premium go?" *JAMA* 317(22): 2269–2270.

Reverby, Susan. (1987). "A caring dilemma: Womanhood and nursing in historical perspective" *Nursing Research* 36(1): 5–11.

Riley, Gerald, and James Lubitz. (2010). "Long-term trends in medicare payments in the last year of life" *Health Services Research* (April) 45(2): 565–576. doi:10.1111/j.1475-6773.2010.01082.x

Roberts, T. (2006). "The history and (and future) of MRI physics" *Medical Physics* 33(6). doi:10.1118/1.2241493

Robinson, Andrew, Kirsten Hohmann, Julie Rifkin, Daniel Topp, Christine Gilroy, Jeffrey Pickard, and Robert Anderson. (2004). "Direct-to-consumer pharmaceutical advertising: Physician and public opinion and potential effects on the physician-patient relationship" *Archives of Internal Medicine* 164(4): 427–432. doi:10.1001/archinte.164.4.427

Robinson, Fiona. (1999). *Globalizing Care: Ethics, Feminist Theory, and International Relations*. Boulder, CO: Westview Press.

Rocker, Carol. (2008). "Addressing nurse-to-nurse bullying to promote nurse retention" *The Online Journal of Issues in Nursing* 13(3). doi:10.3912/OJIN. Vol13No03PPT05

Rodwin, Marc. (2001). "Commentary: The politics of evidence-based medicine" *Journal of Health Politics, Policy, and Law* 26(2): 439–446.

Rothschild, Joan. (2005). *The Dream of the Perfect Child*. Indianapolis: Indiana University Press.

Rowland, Robyn. (1992). *Living Laboratories: Women and Reproductive Technologies*. Indianapolis: Indiana University Press.

Ruddick, Sara. (1989). *Maternal Thinking: Toward a Politics of Peace*. Boston: Beacon Press.

Ryan, Maura. (2003). *Ethics and Economics of Assisted Reproduction: The Cost of Longing*. Washington, DC: Georgetown University Press.

Sackett, David, William Rosenberg, J. A. Muir Gray, R. Brian Haynes, and W. Scott Richardson. (1996). "Evidence-based medicine: What it is and what it isn't." *British Medical Journal* (January 13) 312: 71–72.

Sackett, David, Sharon E. Straus, W. Scott Richardson, William Robinson, and R. Brian Haynes. (2000). *Evidence-Based Medicine: How to Practice and Teach EBM*. London: Churchill Livingstone.

Sanmartin, Claudia, Edward Ng, Debra Blackwell, Jane Gentleman, Michael Martinez, and Catherine Simile. (2004). *Joint Canada/United States Survey of Health 2002–2003*. Atlanta, GA: Authority of the Minister Responsible for Statistics Canada in collaboration with the National Center for Health Statistics, U.S. Centers for Disease Control and Prevention.

Savulescu, Julian. (2001). "Procreative beneficence: Why we should select the best children" *Bioethics* 15(5–6): 413–426.

Sawyer, Bradley, and Cynthia Cox. (2018). "How does health spending in the U.S. compare to other countries?" in Peterson-Kaiser Health System Tracker. Menlo Park, CA: Kaiser Family Foundation.

Schmidt, Volker H. (1998). "Selection of recipients for donor organs in transplant medicine" *Journal of Philosophy and Medicine* 23(1): 50–74.

Schoen, C. and S. Collins. (2017). "The big five health insurers' membership and revenue trends: Implications for public policy" *Health Affairs* 36(12): 2185–2194.

Schoen, C., and M. M. Doty. (2004). "Inequities in access to medical care in five countries: Findings from the 2001 commonwealth fund international health policy survey" *Health Policy* 67(3): 309–322.

Sevenhuisjen, Selma. (2003). "The place of care: The relevance of the feminist ethic of care for social policy" *Feminist Theory* 4(2): 179–197.

Sevenhuisjen, Selma. (2004). *Citizenship and the Ethics of Care: Feminist Considerations on Justice, Morality and Politics*. New York: Routledge.

Shang, Baoping, and Dana Goldman. (2007). "Does age or life expectancy better predict health care expenditures?" *Health Economics* 17(4): 487–501. http://onlinelibrary.wiley.com/doi/10.1002/hec.1295/full

Shanley, Mary Lyndon. (1995). " 'Surrogate mothering' and women's freedom: A critique of contracts for human reproduction" in *Expecting Trouble: Surrogacy,*

Fetal Abuse & New Reproductive Technologies, Patricia Boling, ed. Boulder, CO: Westview Press.

Shapiro, Daniel. (1998). "Why even egalitarians should favor market health insurance" in *Problems of Market Liberalism*, Ellen Frankel Paul, Fred D. Miller, and Jeffrey Paul, eds. Cambridge: Cambridge University Press, pp. 84–132.

Shaviro, Daniel. (2004). *Who Should Pay for Medicare?* Chicago: University of Chicago Press.

Sherwin, Susan. (1992). *No Longer Patient: Feminist Ethics and Health Care*. Philadelphia: Temple University Press.

Shin, David, Lina Poder, Jesse Courtier, David Naeger, Antonio Westphalen, and Fergus Coakley. (2011). "CT and MRI of early intrauterine pregnancy" *American Journal of Roentgenology* (February) 196(2): 325–330.

Siebold, Cathy. (1992). *The Hospice Movement: Easing Death's Pains*. London: Twayne Publishers.

Slote, Michael. (2007). *The Ethics of Care and Empathy*. New York: Routledge.

Sokol, Daniel. (2006). "How the doctor's nose has shortened over time: A historical overview of the truth-telling debate in the doctor-patient relationship. *JRSM* 99(12): 632–636.

Sparrow, Robert. (2005). "Defending deaf culture: The case of cochlear implants" *The Journal of Political Philosophy* 13(2): 135–152.

Spiro, Howard, Mary McCrea Curnen, and Lee Palmer Wandel, eds. (1996). *Facing Death: Where Culture, Religion, and Medicine Meet*. New Haven: Yale University Press.

Sprangers, Mirjam, and Neir Aaronson. (1992). "The role of health care providers and significant others in evaluating the quality of life of patients with chronic disease: A review" *Journal of Clinical Epidemiology* (July) 45(7): 743–760.

Starr, Paul. (1982). *The Social Transformation of American Medicine*. New York: Basic Books.

Steinbock, Bonnie. (1992). *Life Before Birth: The Moral Status of Embryos and Fetuses*. Oxford: Oxford University Press.

Steinorth, Petra. (2011). "Impact of health savings accounts on precautionary savings, demand for health insurance and prevention effort" *Journal of Health Economics* 30(2): 458–465.

Stone, Alison. (2004). "Essentialism and anti-essentialism in feminist philosophy" *Journal of Moral Philosophy* 1(2): 135–153.

Squires, David, and Chloe Anderson. (2015). *U.S. Health Care from a Global Perspective: Spending, Use of Services, Prices and Health in 13 Countries*. New York: The Commonwealth Fund.

Tallman, Ruth. (2018). "Self-governed agency: A feminist approach to patient noncompliance" *International Journal of Feminist Approaches to Bioethics* 11(1): 76–90.

Terry, Gareth, and Virginia Braun. (2011). " 'It's kind of me taking responsibility for these things': Men, vasectomy and 'contraceptive economies'" *Feminism and Psychology* 21(4): 477–495.

Thomas, John, John O'Leary, and Terri Fried. (2009). "Understanding their options: Determinants of hospice discussion for older persons with advanced illness" *Journal of General Internal Medicine* 24(8): 923–928.

Thorne, Sally. (2016). "The status and use value of qualitative research findings" in *Exploring Evidence-Based Practice: Debates and Challenges in Nursing*, Martin Lipscomb, ed. New York: Routledge, pp. 151–164.

Timmermans, Stefan, and Alison Angell. (2001). "Evidence-based medicine, clinical uncertainty, and learning to doctor" *Journal of Health and Social Behavior* 42: 342–359.

Timmermans, Stefan, and Marc Berg. (2003). *The Gold Standard: The Challenge of Evidence-Based Medicine and Standardization in Health Care.* Philadelphia: Temple University Press.

Tonelli, M. (1998). "The philosophical limits of evidence-based medicine" *Academic Medicine* 73(12): 1234–1240.

Tronto, Joan. (1994). *Moral Boundaries: A Political Argument for an Ethic of Care.* New York: Routledge.

Tronto, Joan. (2009). "Consent as a grant of authority: A care ethics reading of informed consent" in *Naturalized Bioethics: Toward Responsible Knowing and Practice.* Cambridge: Cambridge University Press, pp. 182–198.

Tronto, Joan. (2012). "Partiality based on relational responsibilities: Another approach to global ethics" *Ethics and Social Welfare* 6(3): 303–316.

Tronto, Joan. (2013). *Caring Democracy: Markets, Equality, and Justice.* New York: New York University Press.

Tseng, Philip, Robert Kaplan, and Barak Richman. (2018). "Administrative costs associated with Physician billing and insurance-related activities at an academic health care system" *JAMA* 319(7): 691–697.

University of Maryland. (1999). "News release: 'The break-even cost of kidney transplants is shrinking'" www.umm.edu/news/releases/kidcost.htm

Upshur, Ross, and C. Shawn Tracy. (2004). "Legitimacy, authority, and hierarchy: Critical challenges for evidence-based medicine" *Brief Treatment and Crisis Intervention* 4(3): 197–204.

Veatch, Robert. (2002). *The Basics of Bioethics,* 2nd ed. New York: Pearson.

Vosman, Frans. (2017). "The moral relevance of lived experience in coplex hospital practices: A phenomenological approach" in *Theological Ethics and Moral Value Phenomena: The Experience of Values,* Steven van den Heuvel, Patrick Nullens, and Angela Roothman, eds. New York: Routledge, pp. 65–92.

Wagner, Edward. (2000). "The role of patient care teams in chronic disease management" *British Medical Journal* 320(7234): 569–572.

Wagner, Natalie. (2006). "Health care cost comparison of the United States and Canada" *OLR Research Report.* www.cga.ct.gov/2006/rpt/2006-R-0289.htm

Wajman, José Roberto, Sheilla de Medeiros Correia Marin, Paulo Henrique Ferreira Bertolucci, Marcia Lorena Fagunde Chaves, and Theresa Bromley. (2018). "Qualitative features in clinical trials: Coordinates for prevention of passive and active misconduct" *International Journal of Clinical Trials* 5(1): 5–11.

Walker, Margaret Urban. (2009). "Introduction: Groningen naturalism in bioethics" in *Naturalized Bioethics: Toward Responsible Knowing and Practice.* Cambridge: Cambridge University Press, pp. 1–22.

Walling, Anne, Steven Asch, Karl Lorenz, Carol Roth, Tod Barry, Katherine Kahn, and Neil Wenger. (2010). "The quality of care provided to hospitalized patients at the end of life" *Archives of Internal Medicine* 170(12): 1057–1063.

Watson, Jean. (2012). *Human Caring Science: A Theory of Nursing,* 2nd ed. Sudbury, MA: Jones & Bartlett.

Weale, Albert. (1998). "Ethical issues in social insurance for health" in *Health Care, Ethics, and Insurance,* Tom Sorrell, ed. New York: Routledge, pp. 137–150.

Weigle, Matthias, Nicole Stab, Isabel Herms Dip-Psych, Peter Angerer, Winfried Hacker, and Jürgen Glasser. (2016). "The associations of supervisor support and work overload with burnout and depression: A cross-sectional study in two nursing settings" *Journal of American Nursing* 72(8): 1774–1788.

Werblow, Andreas, Stefan Felder, and Peter Zweifel. (2007). "Population ageing and health care expenditure: A school of 'red herrings'?" *Health Economics* 16(10): 1109–1126. http://onlinelibrary.wiley.com/doi/10.1002/hec.1213/full

Widdershoven-Heerding, I. (1987). "Medicine as a form of practical understanding" *Theoretical Medicine* 8(2): 179–185.

Williams, Robin. (2006). "Compressed foresight and narrative bias: Pitfalls in assessing high technology futures" *Science as Culture* 15(4): 327–348.

Winkelmayer, W. C., M. C. Weinstein, M. A. Mittleman, R. J. Glynn, and J. S. Pliskin. (2002). "Health economic evaluations: The special case of end-stage renal disease treatment" *Medical Decision Making* 22(5): 412–430.

Winner, Langdon. (1986). *The Whale and the Reactor: A Search for Limits in an Age of High Technology.* Chicago: University of Chicago Press.

Winterbottom, Anna, Hilary Bekker, Mark Conner, and Andrew Mooney. (2008). "Does narrative information bias individual's decision making? A systematic review" *Social Science and Medicine* 67(123): 2079–2088.

Woolf, Steven, and Russell Harris. (2012). "The harms of screening: New attention to an old concern" *JAMA* 307(6): 565–566.

Woolhandler, Steffie, Terry Campbell, and David Himmelstein. (2003). "Costs of health care administration in the United States and Canada" *New England Journal of Medicine* 349: 768–775.

Wyer, P. C., and S. A. Silver. (2009). "Where is the wisdom? A conceptual history of evidence-based medicine" *Journal of Evaluation in Clinical Practice* 15(6): 891–898.

Young, Joanne. (2011). "Lincoln senator directs attention to prenatal care issue" *Lincoln Journal Star* (March 17).

Index

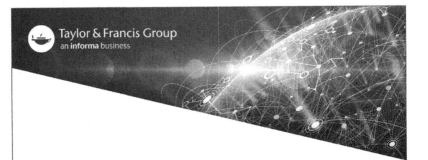

Printed in the United States
by Baker & Taylor Publisher Services